# MR Cholangiopancreatography

Springer-Verlag Berlin Heidelberg GmbH

P. Pavone · R. Passariello

# MR Cholangio-
# pancreatography

Techniques, Results,
and Clinical Indications

With the Collaboration of
A. Laghi and C. Catalano

Foreword by J. T. Ferrucci

With 92 Figures in 191 Separate Illustrations

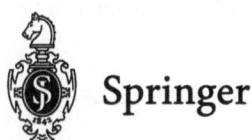 Springer

Paolo Pavone, MD
Professor Roberto Passariello, MD
Andrea Laghi, MD
Carlo Catalano, MD
Università degli Studi di Roma "La Sapienza"
Istituto di Radiologia, Cattedra II
00161 Rome
Italy

ISBN 978-3-642-64416-0       ISBN 978-3-642-60461-4 (eBook)
DOI 10.1007/978-3-642-60461-4

Library of Congress Cataloging-in-Publication Data. Pavone, P. (Paolo) MR
cholangiopancreatography: techniques, results, and clinical indications / P. Pavone, R. Passariello in collaboration with A. Laghi and C. Catalano.    p.    cm.
Includes bibliographical references and index.
        1. Bile ducts–Magnetic resonance imaging. 2. Pancreas–Magnetic re-
sonance imaging. I. Passariello, R. (Roberto), 1942–   . II: Title. [DNLM: 1. Bile
Ducts–pathology. 2. Pancreas–pathology. 3. Magnetic Resonance Imaging–methods. 4. Cholangiography–methods. WI 750 P339m 1997] RC849.P38 1997
616.3'6507548–dc20 DNLM/DLC for Library of Congress 96-30464 CIP

© Springer-Verlag Berlin Heidelberg 1997
Softcover reprint of the hardcover 1st edition 1997

Satz: K+V Fotosatz Beerfelden

SPIN: 10525816       21/3135-5 4 3 2 1 0 – Printed on acid-free paper

# Foreword

The emergence of magnetic resonance cholangiopancreatography (MRCP) has been one of the most rapid radiologic success stories in recent memory. The two major elements of the tale are the imaging radiologic technique and the clinical impact.

MRCP evolved as a result of interactions between fast spin echo pulse sequences, image post processing, especially maximum intensity projections (MIP), and various techniques for motion suppression. Image display formatting white fluid on a black background fortuitously simulated contrast radiography while the two-dimensional projectional image was easier for clinicians to analyze than cross-sectional ultrasound or computed tomography (CT). MRCP also produces a global representation of both the biliary and pancreatic duct systems with associated periductal pathology (cysts, diverticula, fluid collections) which was rarely, if ever, so completely displayed on retrograde endoscopic cholangiopancreatography (ERCP). Several groups noted the added value of analyzing the raw data in source images in addition to the reconstructed MIP images, especially for the detection of calculi. All of the above were quickly recognized by most early investigators, and MRCP research groups flourished in university radiology departments the world over.

The clinical acceptance of MRCP by gastroenterologists and surgeons has surprised even the most seasoned gastrointestinal radiologists. Accurate demonstration of duct calibre, obstruction, calculi, cysts, and diverticula have made MRCP immediately competitive as a diagnostic screening technique for pancreaticobiliary disease. In the biliary tract, anatomic demonstration of obstruction, including the degree of proximal dilatation is often superior to that obtained by ERCP because of the risk of over-injection (sepsis). Accuracy for detection of choledocholithiasis at MRCP now equals that of the more invasive ERCP, making the technique now potentially applicable as a noninvasive

screening technique. Survey screening to detect biliary
duct anomalies before laparoscopic cholecystectomy is another important potential application in the biliary tract.
In the case of pancreatic diseases, detection and follow-up
of complications of pancreatitis, including duct strictures,
calculi, and pseudocysts appears clinically more worth-
while than pancreatic cancer where conventional CT is
quite satisfactory. Anomalies of the pancreatic duct such as
pancreas divisum are also well-demonstrated. Although the
relationship between MRCP and ERCP will continue to
evolve, ERCP obviously has important therapeutic deriva-
tives and the extent to which MRCP can substitute or com-
pliment the diagnostic aspects of ERCP will be influenced
by numerous factors including availability of proper equipment, radiologists' expertise, referring clinicians practice
style, and reimbursement.

The group from The University of Rome "La Sapienza"
was one of the early contributors to this important new development for diagnostic radiologic imaging in the upper
abdomen, and this volume adds significantly to our knowledge of this subject.

Boston, Massachusetts                    Joseph T. Ferrucci, MD

# Acknowledgments

The preparation of a book requires three distinct types of efforts: collection of consistent experimental and clinical material, preparation of the texts, and assembly of texts and pictures in a complete book. By themselves, the authors would have never been able to publish this work without the collective help of a group of enthusiastic people. Among these, the most significant support has come from one of our residents, Valeria Panebianco. She has been at the console until late at night collecting clinical data, as well as pushing us to prepare manuscripts, and preparing and rearranging the material herself. However, we must also acknowledge the very important clinical and editorial contribution of other residents, including A. Messina, R.F. Grasso, A. Scipioni, and L. Broglia. Younger colleagues have also contributed: A. Corsetti, F. Fanelli, F. Assael, S. Pirillo. F. Russo, and A. Grossi were the authors of the illustrations, proving to us that their expertise in imaging goes beyond 'simple' radiology. The chapter on benign stenosis was prepared with the help of M. Di Girolamo, a former resident in our department.

A special acknowledgment goes to our endoscopists, who have supported our efforts from the very beginning. F. Fiocca and E. Grasso are also the authors of the last chapter on the residual role of ERCP.

We wish to thank Prof. D.G. Faroni and Mr. R. Innocenzi of I.N.I. for allowing late-evening activity on the MR system for research purposes and S. Cavalaggio and E. Lucci for precious technical support. The images were reproduced by our expert, S. Genna. L. Contini has helped in the filing of the slide material.

The research project on MRCP is partially supported by the Italian Council for Research (CNR), Progetto Finalizzato ACRO, Sottoprogetto 5.

June 1996                                          Paolo Pavone
                                                   Roberto Passariello

# Contents

# CHAPTER 1

# Imaging Techniques

## Introduction

Several imaging techniques, both invasive and noninvasive, are commonly used for evaluating biliopancreatic ducts: intravenous cholangiography, ultrasound, computed tomography (CT), magnetic resonance (MR), percutaneous transhepatic cholangiography (PTC) and endoscopic retrograde cholangiopancreatography (ERCP). Intravenous cholangiography is limited by the major drawback, namely the lack of opacification of the biliary system, which occurs in 30%–40% of cases. Moreover, in a prospective study intravenous cholangiography was useful in detecting choledocholithiasis only in 1.5% of cases [1, 2]. Risks related to adverse reaction of contrast agent, the cost of the procedure, and the poor anatomical definition of the intra- and extrahepatic bile ducts should be considered if a cost–effectiveness analysis is performed [3]. Ultrasound, CT, and conventional MR are currently used in the initial evaluation of patients with symptoms and signs related to the pancreaticobiliary system. The diagnostic accuracy varies with the various pathologies, but each of the previous techniques, offering an indirect representation of the biliary ducts, is often insufficient to provide a correct diagnosis and basis for treatment of the biliary obstruction [4–6].

Direct cholangiographic views of the biliary tract can only be obtained through invasive techniques, that is, ERCP and PTC. The main advantages of ERCP are high resolution and the possibility of performing a therapeutic procedure immediately after the diagnosis is obtained. Technical limitations can prevent a successful ERCP, such as in the case of hepaticojejunostomy or gastric resection with anastomosis beyond the jejunum [7]. Moreover, operator skill is required in retroperitoneal neoplasms, anomalies in the position of the ampulla of Vater, postoperative modifications (Bilroth II reconstruction), and juxtapapillary duodenal diverticula (50% of patients older than 80 years undergoing ERCP) [8, 9]. In addition, although considered a relatively safe procedure ERCP can present some complications, particularly postpancreatographic acute pancreatitis (asymptomatic hyperamilasemia is observed in 70% of cases whereas acute pancreatitis develops in 0.5% of cases) [10] and cholangitis (1% of patients) [11]. Mortality occurs in about 1% of patients [12]. PTC has the same diagnostic role as ERCP, but it is invasive, risky (sepsis in 1.4%, mortality in 0.20%) [13], and expensive.

Recently the development of fast imaging techniques and the improvement of abdominal image quality have led to magnetic resonance cholangio-pancreatography (MRCP), generating new interest in MR evaluation of biliopancreatic diseases. MRCP is a new diagnostic, noninvasive technique for direct visualization of the biliary ducts with images similar to those of ERCP and PTC. It requires neither contrast medium injection nor any biliary intervention. The optimization of an MRCP sequence requires fast imaging sequences and the availability of other complimentary techniques, such as artifact reduction, fat-suppression, and three-dimensional acquisition.

## Fast Imaging

Fast imaging techniques have been rapidly developing in recent years thanks to technological improvements in hardware and software. The reasons for developing fast imaging are: (a) to increase the number of examinations per unit of time; (b) to minimize patient disconfort; (c) to image severily ill patients; (d) to reduce motion artifacts (from respiration, cardiac pulsation and voluntary motion) by using breath-hold techniques; (e) to perform functional studies (dynamic MRI); and (f) to use three-dimensional (3D) imaging routinely.

Typically the acquisition time for a conventional two-dimensional (2D) MR image is calculated by: $TR \times Ny \times NEX$. To reduce the scan time it is necessary to modify one of the previous three parameters. NEX is the available signal–noise ratio (SNR). The better the SNR is, the smaller the NEX which can be chosen. Of course, when NEX is reduced by half, the scan time is reduced by half, and the SNR is decreased by approximately 40% [14]. The minimum NEX is 1 unless half-Fourier imaging is used. With this technique only 50% of the $k$ space is sampled while the remaining 50% is filled retrospectively based on the mirror-image Hermitian conjugate symmetry of $k$ space [15]. However, for a reduction in artifacts generated by this technique, the $k$ space is sampled slightly more than 50% (Fig. 1). The scan time can be shortened by reducing the phase-encoding steps (Ny) at the expense of a reduced spatial resolution. A good compromise between scan time and spatial resolution can be obtained by using a rectangular matrix (e.g., 256×192). A rectangular field of view (FOV) gives the advantage of mantaining the same matrix with a reduced scan time, but with the disadvantage of a reduced SNR and wrap-around artifacts if the FOV is too small.

The last approach is the reduction in TR. TR is in fact the longest period of time in the pulse sequence, especially in spin echo sequences, where a long time is necessary to recover the longitudinal magnetization following the 90° RF pulse. Therefore reducing TR in a spin echo sequence would be to introduce more and more T1 weighting and to reduce the number of slices when a multislice technique is used. To avoid this problem gradient-recalled echo (GRE) sequences were introduced, where a flip angle smaller than 90° is used and where the signal is obtained by refocusing gradients instead of 180° pulses.

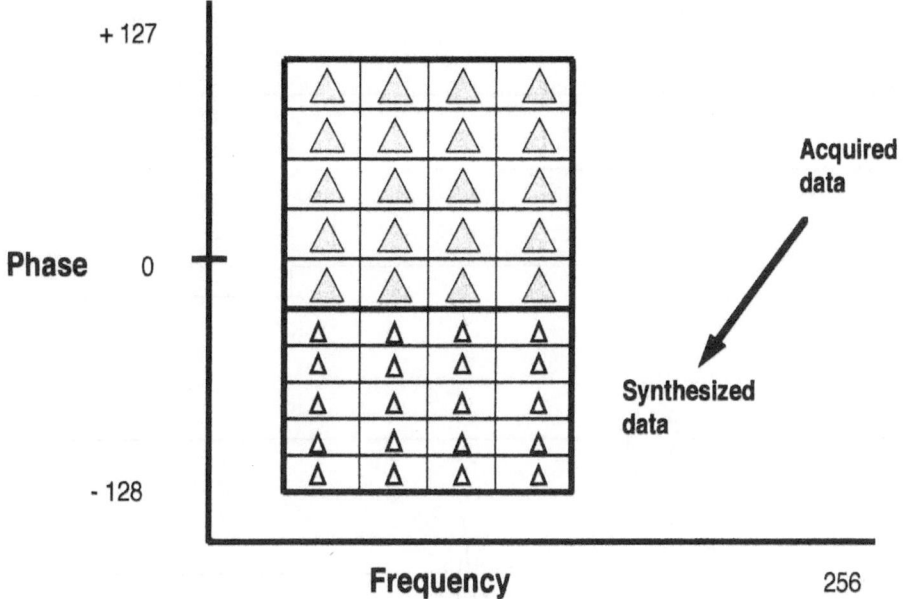

**Fig. 1.** *k* space representation of half-Fourier technique. Slightly more than 50% of data are acquired directly; the remaining data are retrospectively filled on the basis of the mirror-image Hermitian conjugate symmetry of *k* space

## Gradient Echo Sequences

### Basic Gradient Echo Sequence

The basic GRE technique has a structure similar to that of a conventional spin echo sequence except that instead of acquiring an spin echo, the 180° pulse is eliminated, and gradient echo is acquired. The gradient echo is formed by gradient refocusing rather than by RF refocusing. In other words, after an RF pulse with arbitrary flip angle is applied, a negative gradient dephases the spins which are subsequently refocused by a positive gradient; as a consequence they generate an echo, called gradient refocused echo [16, 17] (Fig. 2).

The advantages of GRE sequence are related to the short scan time (seconds instead of minutes), flexible contrast (varied by changing TR, TE, and the flip angle), and higher signal if short TRs are needed [18]. It should be pointed out that gradient refocusing corrects only for phase shifts induced by the gradient itself; phase shift resulting from field inhomogeneities, static tissues susceptibility, and chemical shift are not canceled out. Therefore the gradient echo signal decays according to T2*, depending on both T2 and static magnetic field variations.

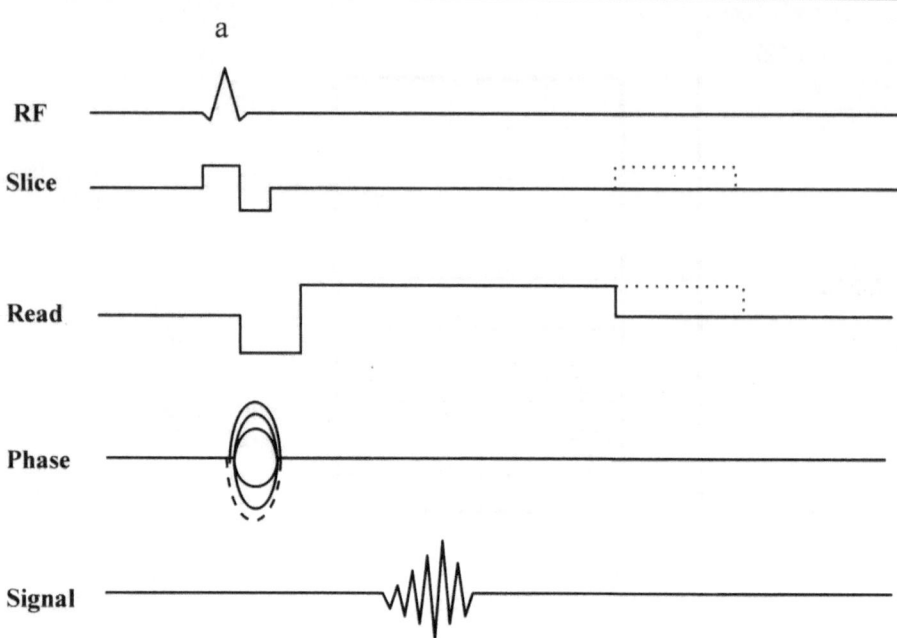

**Fig. 2.** Diagram of GRE sequence. Dephasing gradient pulse produces negative phase shift, while rephasing gradient produces compensatory positive phase shift

### "Modified" Gradient Echo

In fast scan very short TR are used in order to reduce the acquisition time. The fact is that very short TR often result in a TR shorter than the T2 of the tissue being imaged. It determines an image in the steady state, which implies that there is little time for T2 relaxation to occur between excitation pulses [19].

Different GRE techniques have been developed: steady state sampling free induction decay (FID; SS-GRE-FID), which uses residual Mxy rewinder and no spoiler pulse; spoiled GRE (SP-GRE), which adds RF spoiling of residual Mxy; steady state sampling spin echo (SS-GRE spin echo), which uses a long-TE gradient refocused spin echo instead of a gradient refocused FID. In SS-GRE-FID and in spoiled GRE sequences the FID is intentionally dephased to allow for phase encoding and is then rephased immediately via a gradient pulse, which is why these are called gradient recalled pulse sequences. In SS-GRE spin echo sequence a spin echo is created by applying a sequence of RF pulses any two of which can form a spin echo.

### *Steady State Sequence*

These sequences use very short TRs, which result in a steady state condition. To refocus the transversal magnetization they use rewinding gradients. This

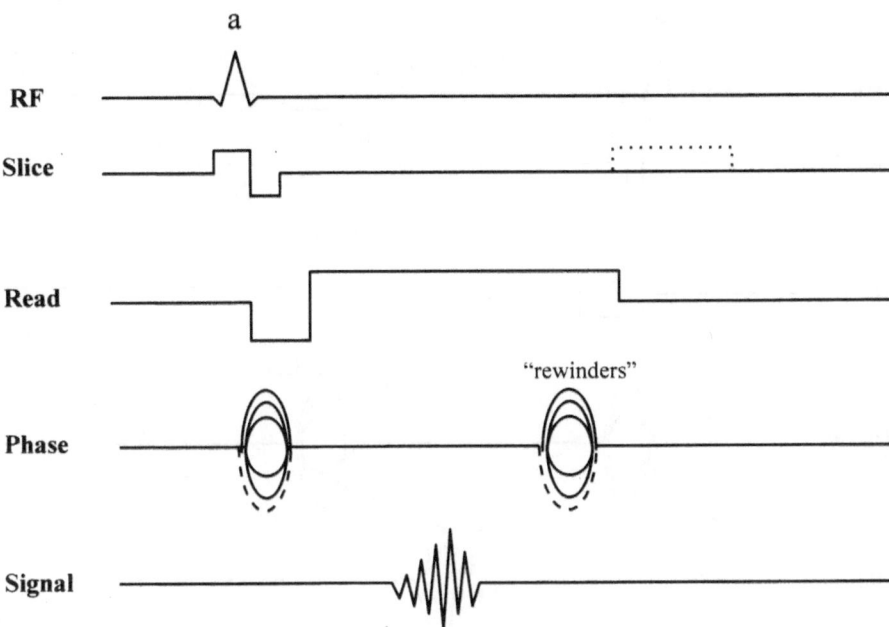

**Fig. 3.** SS-GRE-FID sequence. Phase encoding occurs between the RF excitation and readout of the echo. A rewinder gradient is then applied to preserve residual magnetization on the *xy* plane. It is this rewinder that results in the addition of residual T2 signal to each echo

rewinder preserves the residual transverse magnetization left over from the previous excitations. As a result, this steady state component always makes some contribution to the signal [20–21] (Fig. 3).

### Spoiled GRE Sequence

In these sequences T2 dependence is almost completely eliminated (although T2* is still present) by the disruption of residual transverse component. The term spoiling refers to the purposeful disruption of the buildup of a steady state by using "spoiler" gradients, random RF pulse phases, and variable TR, depending on the different manufacturers [20, 22] (Fig. 4).

Both SS-GRE-FID sequence and spoiled GRE are very sensitive to magnetic susceptibility artifacts, chemical shift artifacts, and image degradation caused by magnetic field inhomogeneities. These artifacts are aggravated by large voxels and long TEs. Obtaining heavily T2-weighted images of good quality is therefore very difficult using these sequences.

### Steady State Sampling Spin Echo

SS-GRE spin echo is the pulse sequence of choice when heavily T2-weighted images are needed. This sequence samples the spin echo rather than a FID

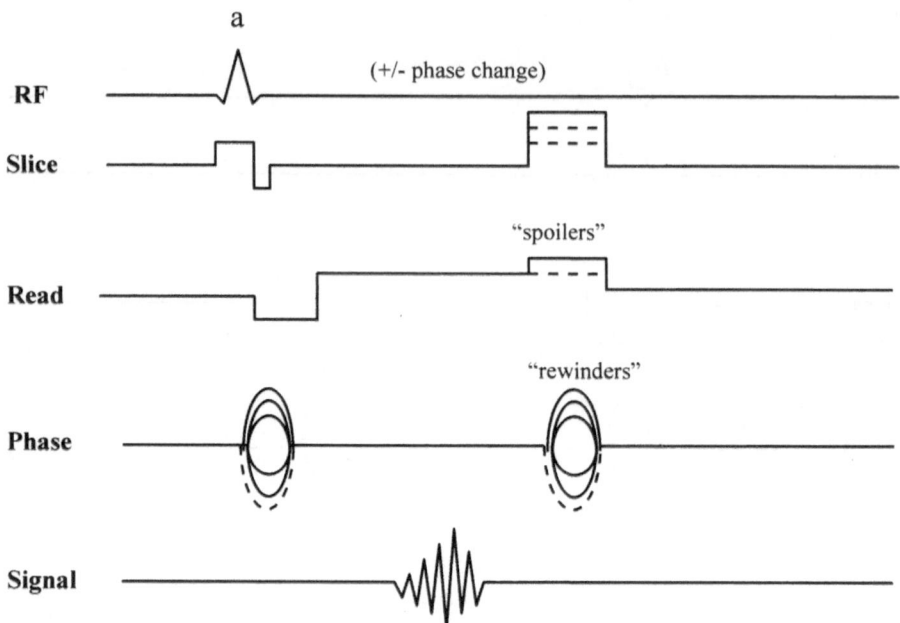

**Fig. 4.** Spoiled GRE. The only difference between the spoiled GRE and the SS-GRE-FID sequence is the spoiled GRE phase offset pulse

signal. The basic principles are as follows: When adding an RF pulse, the main effect is to tilt the longitudinal magnetization and in a limited way to partially refocus the spins on the transverse plane. The second pulse thus has a main component tilting the longitudinal magnetization on the transverse plane and a secondary component refocusing the spins on the transverse plane. The refocused spins generate an echo which can be detected (Fig. 5). The difference between the echo and the FID is that, between the end of the FID and the generation of an echo, T2 decay has occurred, just as in conventional imaging. In contrast to spin echo images, the pulse refocusing the spins is not a dedicated pulse but the following pulse generating the tilting of the longitudinal magnetization. As a consequence it would be impossible to send an RF pulse and at the same time to listen to the echo signal. Thus a gradient to shift the formation of the echo is usually applied. This gradient refocusing determines some sensitivity to susceptibility and chemical shift artifacts as well as inhomogeneities effects [19, 21].

SS-GRE spin echo are the most useful sequences to obtain heavily T2-weighted images with gradient echo technique; they are not so sensitive to magnetic susceptibility and chemical shift artifacts as the other GRE sequences; the main limitations are related to increased sensitivity to factors disrupting the steady state (flow, respiratory motion) and the low SNR when long TEs are used.

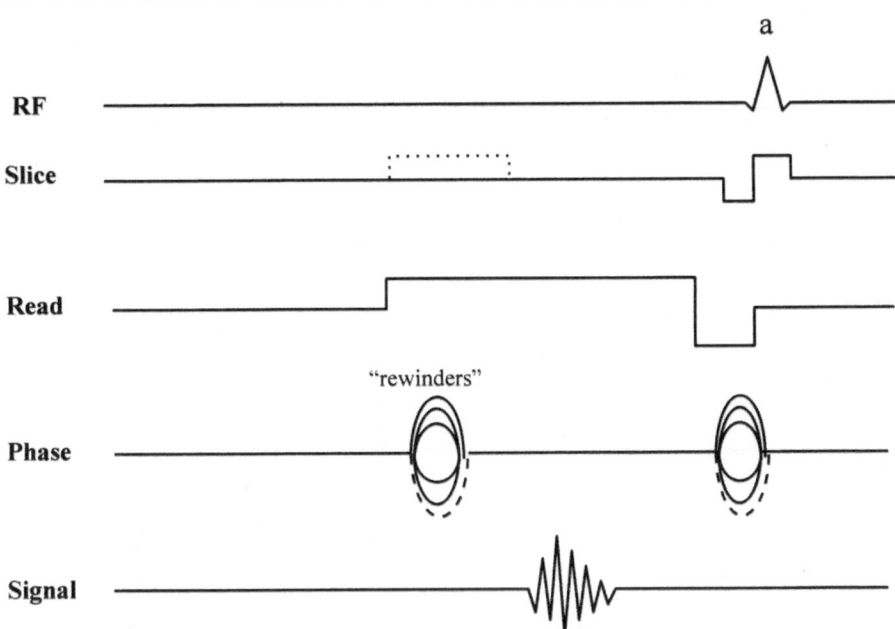

**Fig. 5.** SS-GRE spin echo sequence. When adding an RF pulse, the main effect is to tilt the longitudinal magnetization and in a limited way to partially refocus the spins on the transverse plane. Thus the second pulse has a main component tilting the longitudianl magnetization on the transverse plane and a secondary component refocusing the spins on the transverse plane. The refocused spins generates an echo which can be detected

### Rapid GRE

Rapid GRE sequences require fast sampling time and rapid ramping of the gradients, both available on new commercial equipments. If very short TR values are used, a steady state cannot be fully established, and as a consequence loss of image resolution can occur as well as poor image contrast. However, the main advantage of these sequences is that they are suitable for breath-hold abdominal studies and for dynamic contrast-enhanced studies (perfusion studies) [23, 24].

The poor tissue contrast has been restored by the development of the so-called magnetization-prepared GREs. They consist of two independent modules: a preparation module and a data acquisition module. The preparation module can be modified in order to obtain T1 or T2 contrast, as well as to suppress fat signal by adding a chemical shift selective prepulse [25, 26] (Fig. 6).

## Fast Spin Echo Technique

Fast spin echo sequences are recently developed modifications of the rapid acquisition relaxation enhanced (RARE) sequences, originally introduced

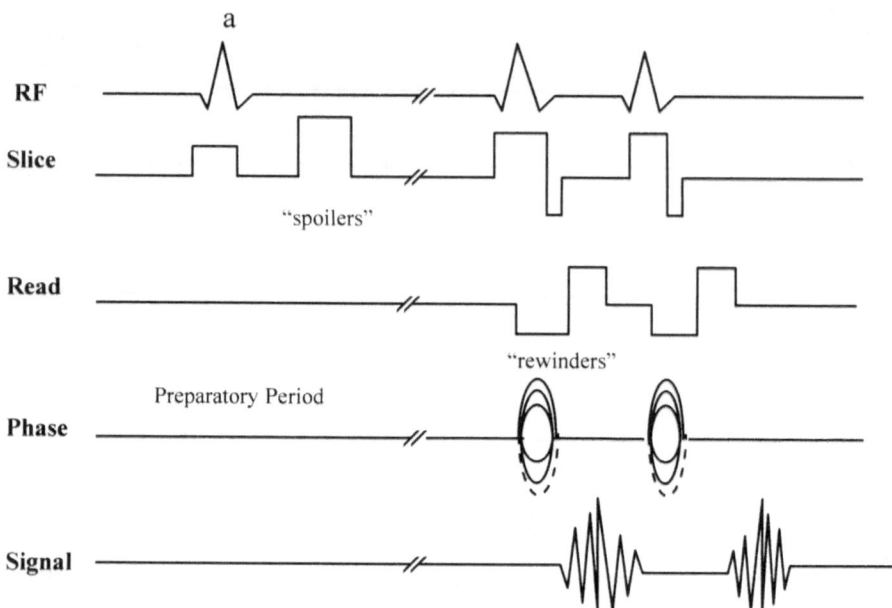

**Fig. 6.** Magnetization prepared GRE sequence. It consists of two independent modules: a preparation module and a data acquisition module. The preparation module can be modified to obtain T1 or T2 contrast, as well as to suppress fat signal by adding a chemical shift selective prepulse

over 30 years ago [27, 28]. In RARE and in fast spin echo imaging a series of spin echo images are generated using repeated 180° pulses; each echo is phase-encoded with a distinct phase-encoding gradient, readout in the presence of a frequency-encoding gradient, and phase "unwound" after readout [29, 30]. The turbo spin echo method combines the acquisition of multiple $k$ profiles per excitation with the multiple slice technique. Each 90° RF pulse is followed by a series of 180° refocusing pulses, generating multiple echoes, resulting in corresponding number of profiles. Each group of pulses/profiles is defined "shot." The shots are acquired at regular intervals (TR) until the image is complete. The number of refocusing pulses and consequently echoes is referred to as turbo factor or echo train length (ETL; Fig. 7).

Turbo spin echo sequences allow a twofold to several-fold reduction in acquisition time compared with conventional spin echo sequences. For example, for a conventional spin echo with the parameters of TR=2000, matrix=256×256, NEX=2, the acquisition time is about 17 min. In contrast, a T2-weighted turbo spin echo with the same parameters lasts about 1.7 min, a tenfold reduction in acquisition time. Theoretically, only one excitation pulse followed by 256 refocusing pulses could be applied, but since in the generation of the multiple echoes a progressive decrease in the signal occurs, only 3–128 echoes (ETL) can be generated in practice.

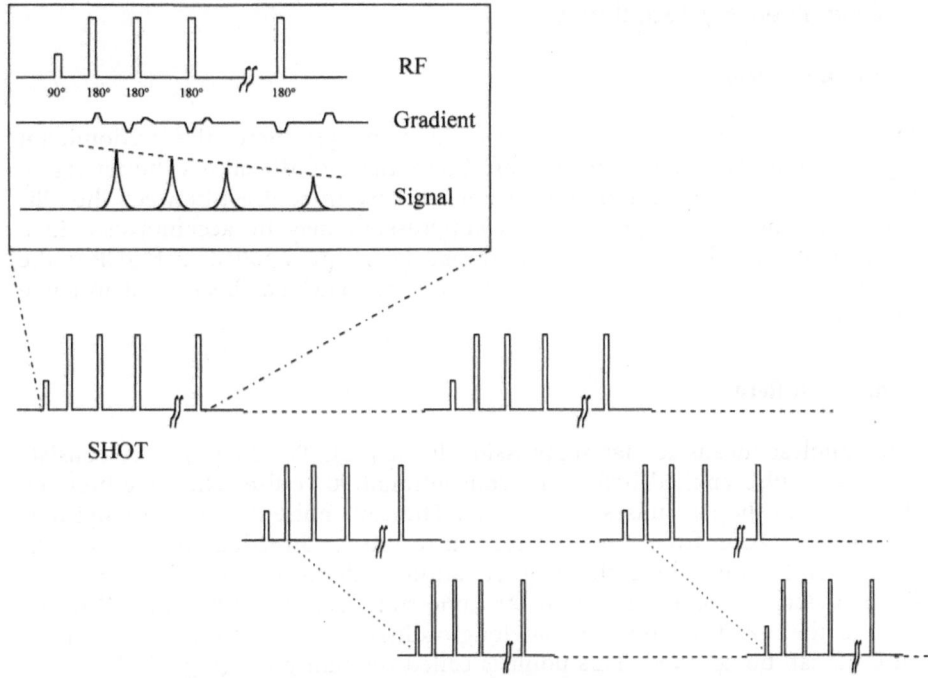

**Fig. 7.** Turbo spin echo sequence. Each 90° RF pulse is followed by a series of 180° refocusing pulses, generating multiple echoes. Each group of pulses/profiles is defined "shot," acquired at regular intervals (TR) until the image is complete

The main advantage of fast spin echo sequences is fast imaging, as we noted above; in addition to reducing the acquisition time, fast imaging can be used to modify other parameters of the sequence to obtain high-quality images. In particular, a higher number of excitations and an increase in matrix size can be selected. Further advantages include fewer motion artifacts and decreased magnetic susceptibility effects when imaging metallic objects and versatility.

Turbo spin echo sequences are particularly useful when acquiring T2-weighted images to obtain high quality T2-weighted images, with contrast similar to conventional T2-weighted spin echo, with reduced motion artifacts, in a fraction of the time needed for a conventional spin echo [31]. The main difference between a conventional T2-weighted spin echo and a T2-weighted turbo spin echo is based on the high signal intensity of fat in the latter. The bright appearance of fat could be a problem, especially when imaging the abdomen, but fat saturation techniques may overcome this limitation.

## Complimentary Techniques

### Fat Suppression

Evaluation of turbo spin echo T2-weighted images shows the predominant signal in the abdomen to be that of abdominal fat. MR allows the fat signal to be canceled, thus obtaining a further increase in contrast between the biliary ducts and the background. Fat suppression may be accomplished in a number of ways, but the most widespread technique applied in MRCP is the chemsat technique, although inversion recovery (IR) has been used in some reports.

### Inversion Recovery

The simplest means for fat suppression is IR [32]. The IR sequence consists of a 180° pulse applied before the conventional 90° pulse. The time between the 180° and the 90° pulses is called TI. The 180° pulse inverts the longitudinal magnetization from the +Z direction to the –Z direction. When the excitation pulse is turned off, the magnetization tends to return towards its equilibrium state in the +Z direction. At same time it crosses from the –Z direction to the +Z direction, and no longitudinal magnetization, either on +Z and –Z, can be detected. This point is called the null point (Fig. 8). As a consequence, selecting an adequate TI results in cancelation of the signal from a tissue. The null point occurs at a time that is about 69% of tissue T1. For example, fat has a T1 of approximately 250 ms and the null point is 160–170 ms. Therefore to suppress fat the TI should be between 160 and 170 ms.

### Chemsat

With this technique a frequency selective presaturation pulse is applied to fat immediately before the excitation pulse, destroying the longitudinal magnetization of the fat [33]. When the excitation pulse is applied, there will not have been sufficient time for longitudinal recovery, and therefore there is little or no magnetization to "move" into the transverse plane. This technique requires that the saturation pulses affect only fat tissues for fat suppression. At 1.5 T hydrogen protons in fat precess at a frequency about 220 Hz lower than those of water. This property, called chemical shift, lets us select the correct center frequency and bandwidth of the saturation pulse such that it affects primarily fat (Fig. 9). To work effectively and consistently throughout the imaging volume, however, a very homogeneous static magnetic field and RF magnetic field are needed. Thus the further away from isocenter, the less effective the saturation is likely to be. This technique is therefore best used with moderate to small FOVs and moderate to small volumes.

In conclusion, fat suppression techniques may offer increased contrast, especially between bile ducts and liver parenchyma, and perhaps a reduction in motion artifacts arising from fatty tissues.

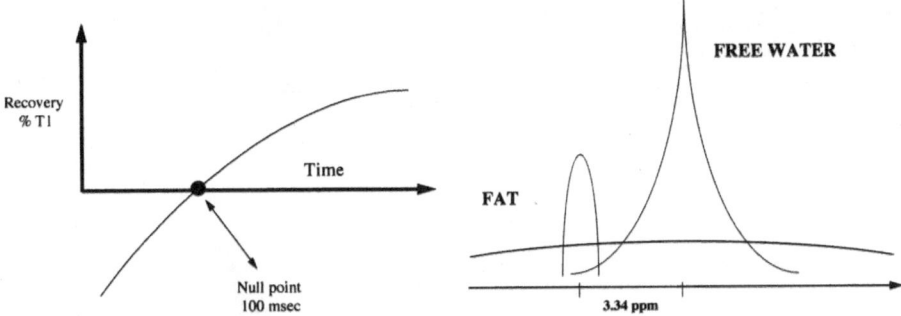

**Fig. 8.** The "null point" associated with the inversion recovery pulse sequence – the point where longitudinal magnetization moves from the –Z to the +Z direction

**Fig. 9.** Chemsat technique. Illustration of the spectral frequency relationship of hydrogen protons in fat and water. At 1.5 T fat precesses about 3.34 ppm slower than water

## Artifact Reduction

Motion artifacts are the most important cause of image degradation, especially in abdominal MR images. The motion that degrade abdominal MR images usually include respiration, blood flow, and gastrointestinal peristalsis [34, 35].

Respiratory motion causes ghost artifacts, loss of tissue intensity, and unsharpness. The use of respiratory triggering allows better image quality. When respiratory triggering is used, data acquisition is started at the end of expiration, and the data for the various slabs are acquired between respiratory excursions, when motion is at minimum. This process is continued until all $k$ space is acquired. This method reduces artifacts at the expense of additional acquisition time and does not work well with irregular breathing. Other techniques such as ordered phase encoding and gradient moment nulling can be employed to reduce motion artifacts [36].

Blood flow artifacts are very common and are usually related to vessels liyng perpendicular to the imaging plane. Several techniques are available for reducing flow artifacts. Spatial presaturation is based on RF pulses applied outside the imaging volume with the aim of destroying the longitudinal magnetization of inflowing spins. The presaturation method has the advantage that it is compatible with most pulse sequences and imaging hardware, and the only disadvantage is the small amount of additional time required within the pulse sequence to apply presaturation pulses (Fig. 10).

Another technique is gradient moment nulling, also called flow compensation [37, 38]. This is used to reduce phase shift phenomena caused by motion and to avoid the intravascular phase dispersion. A series of repeated and inverted gradients are applied; the effect is a phase shift which is equal, but of opposite sign, to that produced by blood flow. In this way signal from blood vessels is reobtained (Fig. 11). This technique has been particularly successful for reducing flow artifacts in gradient echo images, but it is less useful for eliminating flow artifacts in spin echo images. In fact, in a spin

**Fig. 10.** Spatial presaturation
slab selectively eliminates
the signal of flowing blood

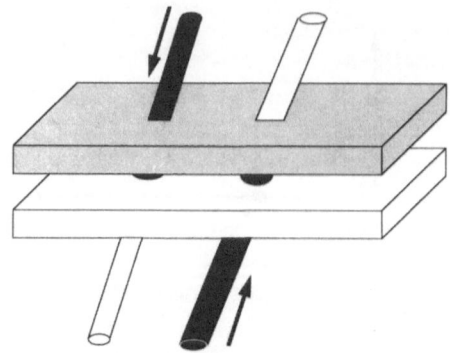

echo sequence mechanisms of wash-in and wash-out are responsible for flow
artifacts, in addition to phase dispersion, and these are not addressed by gradient moment nulling. In some cases a paradoxical increase in artifacts can
be produced by using gradient moment nulling during a spin echo acquisition probably due to the increased peak vascular signal generated by the
elimination of intravoxel phase dispersion.

   In regard to gastrointestinal peristalsis, the approach to date has focused
on prevention, by pharmacological intervention (i.e., antiperistaltic drugs) or
faster imaging techniques [39].

## Three-Dimensional Imaging

With the advent of efficient steady state pulse sequences for MRI, 3D acquisi-
tions have become a practical diagnostic tool for many applications [40, 41].
In 3D techniques, one large volume is excited and then imaged in contiguous

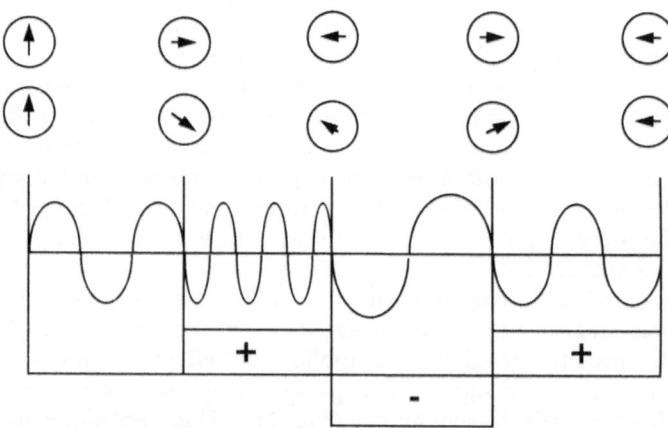

**Fig. 11.** Gradient moment nulling (flow compensation). The phase shift between stationary
and flowing spins is canceled when particular gradient waveforms are employed

slices by using an additional phase-encoding table in the slice direction (Fig. 12). An important advantage of 3D imaging is that it allows very thin slices to be obtained (2–3 mm) using moderate gradient strength. Thinner slices improve spatial resolution with a better definition of small structures (i.e., small stones). The small voxel size also reduces the sensitivity to susceptibility artifacts, a very important factor when dealing with gradient echo sequences. Furthermore, the 3D data sets can be postprocessed using different algorithms, and the images can be reconstructed along different planes. The main limitation is the longer acquisition time, because the scan time is given by: TR×Ny×Nz×Nex. The recent availabiliy of fast imaging techniques has produced a renewed interest in 3D techniques [42].

## MR Cholangiopancreatography

The technique of MRCP is based on heavily T2-weighted pulse sequences, which results in a dramatic increase in contrast between stationary fluids (the bile) and the background (hepatic and pancreatic parenchymas, peritoneal fat). As a result the bile appears at very high signal intensity and the background at low. In addition, no signal comes from flowing blood. Differ-

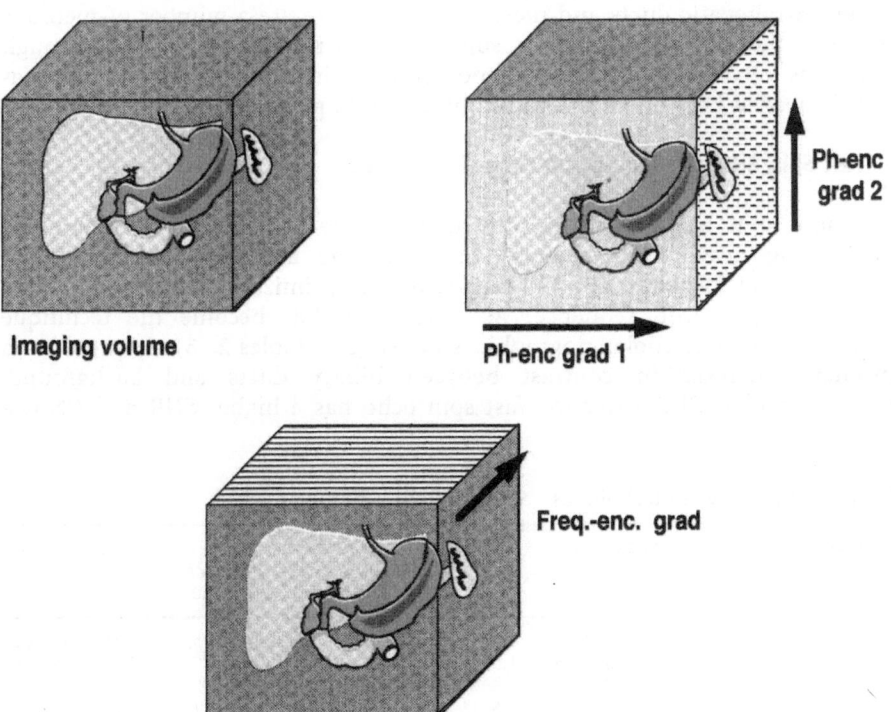

**Fig. 12.** Three-dimensional acquisition. One large volume is excited and the imaged in contiguous slices by using an additional phase-encoding table in the slice direction

ent techniques have been used by the various authors, initially based on gradient echo sequences, but more recently fast spin echo techniques have been more widely used.

### Gradient Echo Techniques

Wallner [43] first described a 2D T2-weighted gradient echo sequence using steady state free precession (SSFP) during breath-hold to produce images of the biliary ducts. The sequence was subsequently optimized by Morimoto [44] by using a 3D acquisition volume and has been evaluated by other authors [45–47] (see Table 1). The SSFP technique is very sensitive to slow flow (in the order of 1 mm/s) along the direction of the read gradient [21]. Under such conditions signal from blood flow is eliminated almost completely. On the other hand, fluid in the steady state is displayed as extremely high-intensity signal. Limitations currently recognized in SSFP sequence are the lack of visualization of small nondilated bile ducts and the Wirsung duct and the lack of evidence of the stricture itself. The high sensitivity to susceptibilty artifacts and as a consequence surgical clips in the volume of examination can cause substantial signal dropout in the image. Nevertheless, contrast between dilated ducts and background liver tissues is high, and intraabdominal fat has relatively high signal intensity and reduces contrast between extrahepatic ducts and mesenteric fat. There are a number of methods that can potentially be used to suppress fat with this sequence, although none has yet been successfully demonstrated. Finally, the patient's cooperation is needed because of a required breath-hold period of 20–40 s.

### Fast Spin Echo Sequences and Other Techniques

The fast spin echo sequence was demonstrated to be very suitable for performing heavily T2-weighted studies in the abdomen in 1993, when Outwater and Meakem [48, 49] proposed the optimization of a non-breath-hold fast spin echo sequence. As a result it has become the technique of choice for MR cholangiographic studies (see Tables 2, 3). It provides a dramatic increase in contrast between biliary ducts and background. Compared with GRE sequence, fast spin echo has a higher SNR and CNR, a

**Table 1.** Gradient echo techniques

| Reference | Sequence | Magnetic field | Parameters TR/TE/FA/NEX/FOV/ Thk (mm)/scan time | Notes |
|-----------|----------|----------------|---------------------------------------------------|-------|
| Wallner 1991 [43] | 2D SSFP | 1.5 | 17/7/70°/3/320–450/5/12″ | BH; body coil |
| Morimoto 1992 [44] | 2D CE-FAST | 1.5 | 17/7/90°/3/350/6/16″ | BH; body coil |
|  | 3D CE-FAST |  | 17/7/90°/1/350/4/20″ |  |
| Ishizaki 1993 [45] | CE-FAST | 1.5 | – | BH |
| Hall-Craggs 1993 [46] | 3D PSIF | 1.0 | 17/7/90°/1/450/3/20″ | BH; body coil |
| Reinhold 1985 [47] | 3D SSFP | 1.5 |  |  |

lower sensitivity to susceptibility artifacts which is very common when studying the biliary tract (i.e., surgical clips, intestinal gas), and a lower sensitivity to motion artifact and blood flow. Moreover, fast spin echo takes advantage of new techniques able to improve the image quality, such as gradient moment nulling, which reduces artifacts from periodic motion, respiratory triggering, and fat suppression to improve the contrast between bile ducts and background. Both breath-hold and non-breath-hold techniques have been developed.

**Table 2.** Fast spin echo techniques

| Reference | Sequence | Magnetic field | Parameters TR/TE/ETL/ NEX/FOV/Thk (mm)/ scan time | Notes |
|---|---|---|---|---|
| Meakem, Outwater 1993 [48, 49] | 2D FSE | 1.5T | 4000/160/16/4/240–280/ 3/8'30" | Non-BH; multicoil |
| Takehara 1994 [50] | 2D FSE | 1.5T | 9000–11000/272/32/1/ 160–200/3/36–44" | BH; surface coil |
| Guibaud 1994 [51] | 2D FSE | 1.5T | 8000/144/16/1–2/340–440/ 3/1'04" | BH (6pts); non-BH (4 pts) |
| Reinhold 1995 [47] | 2D FSE | 1.5T | 8000/144/32/4/340–480/3/ 6'16" | Non-BH; phased-array torso multicoil; high-resolution parameters (512×256) |
| Macaulay 1995 [57] | 2D TSE | 1.5T | 4000/180/29/6/86/3/7'44" | Non-BH |
| Barish, Soto 1995 [14, 28] | 3D FSE | 1.5T | 5000/240/31/1/240/2/10'36" | Non-BH; body coil; coronal and axial plane |
| Pavone, Laghi 1995 [59, 60] | 3D FSE | 0.5T | 3000/700/128/4(6)/240/3/ 4'24" (5'48") | Non-BH; body coil |

**Table 3.** Other techniques

| Reference | Sequence | Magnetic field | Parameters TR/TE/ETL-IR/ NEX/FOV/Thk (mm)/scan time | Notes |
|---|---|---|---|---|
| Laubenberger 1995 [53] | Single-shot RARE | 1.0T | –/998/256/240–500/ 80–500/1–4" | BH; no MIP reconstruction |
| Shiono 1995 [52] | Fast inversion recovery | 1.5T | 3000/350/120 (inversion time)/1/270/40/18" | BH; fat-sat with STIR technique |
| Zuo 1995 [54] | 2D CPMG-like RARE | 1.5T | –/435–800/128–192 (ETL)/ 320–380/5/11–15" | BH; body phased-array coil |
| Wielopolski 1995 [55] | 3D RARE and segmented EPI | 1.5T | 2500–3500/514/190×380/ 2.0–3.5/18–25" | BH; phased-array coil |
| Sananes 1995 [56] | HASTE | 1.0T | 9.2/128/400/5/16" | BH; coronal and axial planes |

## Breath-Hold Techniques

Several authors have explored the possibility of optimizing a breath-hold technique for MR cholangiography [47, 50, 51]. Takehara [50] proposed a breath-hold fast spin echo technique with long ETL (32) using an appropriate surface coil and small FOVs in order to increase SNR. Advantages in using a surface coil are the elimination of the undesirable resonance outside the FOV and a signal increase inside the FOV. Each of these factors allow the use of smaller FOVs with a higher spatial resolution, also during a breath-hold study. The first limitation of this study is the long breath-hold period needed (44 s), which requires oxygen support in elderly patients or segmentation of the images, with the result of poor-quality image reconstructions. The second limitation is the surface coil, which cannot be used in patients in whom the pancreas is too far from the coil; in their series Takehara et al. [50] were able to study all patients thanks to the weight loss secondary to pancreatitis, but they were also studying a Japanese population which has a morphotype very different from that of Western populations.

In the series of Guibaud [51] a breath-hold of more than 1 min was required; patients were asked to hyperventilate for 10 min before they entered the scanner and were given oxygen during the entire examination. In patients unable to take their breath, an examination with two excitations was performed during quiet breathing. Reinhold [47] demonstrated the superiority of 2D fast spin echo sequences over 3D SSFP pulse sequences in detecting both the dilated and nondilated biliary ducts and the pancreatic ducts. Finally, Shiono [52] proposed a breath-hold technique (18 s) using a fast inversion recovery sequence. The advantage is a more homogenous saturation of fat signal than with chemical selective fat saturation pulse.

More recent developments of MR cholangiography are based on different acquisition techniques. Laubenberger [53] reported his experience with a single-shot RARE technique with the acquisition of a single thick slice covering the entire imaging volume within a 4-s breath-hold. The major disadvantage of this technique is the lack of image postprocessing, resulting in the individual tomographic sections not being able to be evaluated. The impact of this on the diagnosis of small structures (i.e., small stones) must be evaluated.

Zuo et al. [54] developed a 2D Carr–Purcell–Meiboom–Gill-like (CPMG-like) RARE multislice sequence and compared it to a 3D PSIF (mirrored fast imaging with steady state precession) gradient echo method and a thick slice single-shot non-breath-hold technique. The results demonstrated that the 2D CPMG-like RARE multislice sequence was able to provide good image quality and acceptable imaging speed, especially if a long effective TE (>650 ms) was employed to obtain a complete decay of the signal of tissue in liver region. The major disadvantages of the other techniques were as follows: 3D PSIF required subjects to maintain a relatively long breath-hold (>22 s) and the images were more susceptible to motions; the non-breath-hold single-shot technique, although providing an overview of the biliary system, could not provide small details for diagnostic purpose due to the lack of maximum intensity projection (MIP) postprocessing.

Wielopolski [55] demonstrated the feasibility of a 3D RARE sequence using segmented echo planar imaging (EPI) readouts on a standard 1.5-T magnet. MR cholangiograms of diagnostic quality were obtained on both healthy volunteers and patients with complete background suppression and good coverage of the region of interest within a single breath-hold of 18–25 s. Further developments of this technique are expected with enhanced gradient rise times and the addition of half Fourier imaging. Finally, Sananes [56] explored the feasibility of MR cholangiography using a half Fourier acquisition single-shot turbo spin echo (HASTE) sequence with a 2-s breath-hold per slice.

### Non-Breath-Hold Techniques

Non-breath-hold techniques sequences were first presented by Outwater [48] and Meakem et al. [49] in 1993. Since then other authors have explored the possibility of MRCP performed during quiet breathing. Non-breath-hold techniques are investigated because most patients are elderly and noncooperative, and they cannot hold their breath for 20–40 s, as required by most of the available breath-hold techniques. Moreover, misregistration artifacts are avoided, and as it is also possible to obtain images with larger matrix size.

Non-breath-hold techniques are all based on fast spin echo sequences. Both 2D and 3D acquisition techniques have been employed. Macaulay [57] and Reinhold [47] explored the potential advantages of a 2D fast spin echo technique, whose main limitation is the slice thickness which cannot be less than 3 mm due to gradient restrictions, with a consequently limited resolution. However, the 3D fast spin echo technique optimized by Barish et al. [58] at 1.5 T, and by Pavone et al. [59, 60] at 0.5 T may overcome these limitations. The use of 3D acquisition improves the SNR and spatial resolution and thus allows use of the body coil. Near isotropic resolution allows MIP images in any plane as well as multiplanar reformatting.

### Personal Experience

In our institution all MRCP examinations are performed using a 0.5-T superconductive magnet with gradient strength of 15 mT/m. We have observed no difference to examinations performed with high field strength equipments. The body coil is used for both excitation and signal reception. We have optimized a 3D, fat-suppressed (SPIR) turbo spin echo sequence with the following imaging parameters: TR=3000 ms, TE=700 ms, ETL=128. Images are obtained on the coronal plane with a 3-mm section thickness and no interslice gap. The imaging volume is positioned to image both the pancreatic and the biliary ducts using as scout view a T2-weighted turbo spin echo sequence acquired on the axial plane. A FOV of 240 mm allows imaging only of the region of interest, avoiding fluid structures from other organs (stomach, duodenum, etc.) which could alter image reconstruction.

The image matrix size is 83×128, but recently a higher resolution technique has been optimized with a 184×256 matrix and the same imaging parameters, except the scan time that is doubled. Even with a reduced matrix size, the image quality is always of diagnostic value, even in very small stones (5 mm). Thus a higher matrix is used only if very detailed images are required (for example, in case of evaluation of secondary pancreatic ducts). Four to six signals are selected for all images with a corresponding acquisition time of 4 min 24 s (5 min 48 s for six averages) for 20 slices. The very short acquisition time is obtained thanks to the elevated turbo factor (128), which allows the data of the sequence to be obtained during a single excitation pulse. Signal loss, compared with a sequence with a lower turbo factor, is not observed.

Respiratory triggering is used for all images to reduce motion artifacts. With respiratory triggering the data are acquired between end expiration and the beginning of the next inspiratory phase. No patient preparation or sedation is required. We prefer to administer antiperistaltic drugs (Buscopan i.m. 20 mg) to reduce motion artifacts resulting from peristalsis and tap water (around 200 cc) in order to obtain a complete filling and visualization of the duodenum.

## Image Reconstruction Techniques

Image reconstruction with projections is performed at the console after all single slices have been acquired, either with 2D or 3D techniques. Different reconstruction techniques can be used: MIP, partial volume reformatting, and volume-rendering techniques.

### Maximum Intensity Projection

MIP was the first reconstruction technique to be developed, and it is still the most used [61, 62]. First the plane of reconstruction (horizontal, vertical, or oblique) must be selected. Then a straight line (ray) is projected through the slices, pixel by pixel, along the selected orientation. The ray passes through the slices and memorizes only the value of maximum intensity, so that the background tissues are canceled. As in all acquired slices, the brightest signal is that of bile and the lowest that of background; therefore this technique enhances all bile duct structures with a canceled signal of background in the reconstructed image (Fig. 13). This procedure is repeated using parallel rays, and angiograms can thus be reconstructed in multiple views. The purpose is to better evaluate bile ducts strictures, also reducing problems related to ducts overlapping. In conventional cholangiography only a limited number of projections can be acquired since each one would require a contrast injection, but with MIP one can obtain an infinite number of projections. Practically, considering that each projection requires high elaboration capabilities and time, image reconstructions are performed every 3°–5°.

Projection images obtained at small intervals can be evaluated either on films or with a cine-display mode. Animation is obtained by quickly presenting on the monitor all the projected images, with consequent rotation of the bile ducts along the selected orientation. This allows a marked improvement in diagnosis with MRCP, through a depth effect and 3D vision. Furthermore, with MRCP it is possible to obtain views different from those usually per-

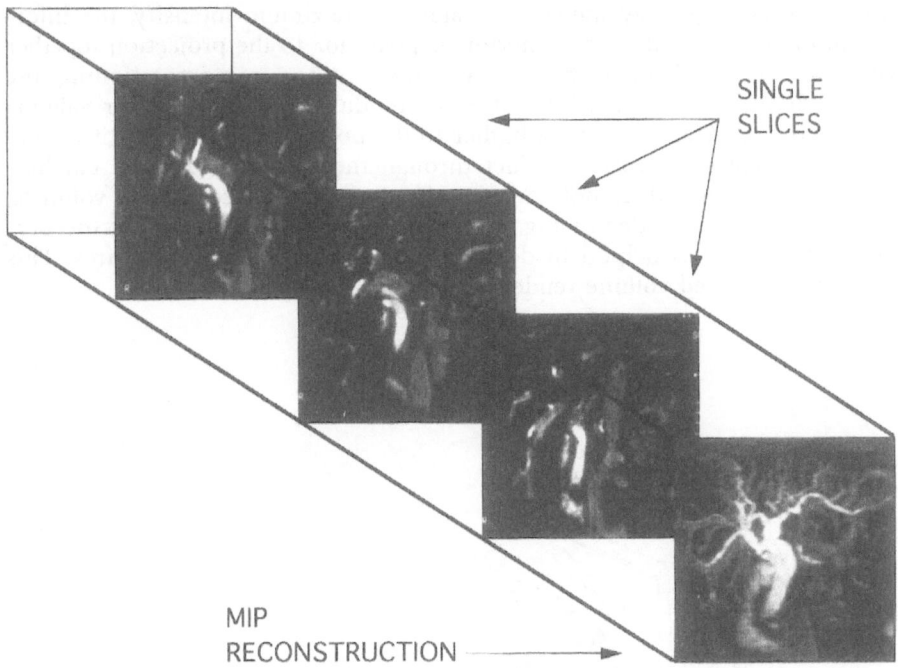

**Fig. 13.** Maximum intensity projection. Multiple parallel rays are projected throuh the volume, considering only the structures with the maximum intensity

formed in conventional cholangiography. Usually MIP reconstruction is obtained on the coronal plane with multiple rotation at 10°–15°. Some authors prefer to obtain axial reconstruction, especially for evaluation of the Wirsung duct. The reconstruction along different angles is very useful in differentiating the anatomical and pathological structures and in evaluating the relationships between them. MIP reconstruction can cancel very small intraductal structures (i.e., small stones), well evident on source images. Thus it is very important the evaluation of the source images ("single slices") for a correct diagnosis, as discussed below.

### Volume Rendering Technique

Single images reconstructed with MIP are not useful concerning image depth. If bile ducts overlapping is present, it is impossible to distinguish which of the two ducts is anterior. Only by viewing images on multiple projections or with the cine mode can a 3D effect be obtained. Unfortunately, the animation display is not always applicable, epecially because it is time consuming.

More recently new reconstruction algorithms that maintain depth information have been developed [63, 64]. The technique is the same of MIP: multiple parallel rays are projected through all the slices acquired. In this case, however, if the ray meets two values of maximum intensity, the information of spatial localization anterior or posterior to the projection together with that of signal intensity is maintained. When reconstructioning the images, the values of signal intensities are modulated so that a lower value is given to the anterior duct and a higher to the posterior; in this way it is possible to visualize the posterior duct through the anterior (Fig. 14). Furthermore, the technique does not consider the ducts as surfaces but as volumes, creating the effect by decreasing the ducts signal intensity towards the periphery. The result is helpful in detecting overlapping biliary structures. This technique is termed volume rendering.

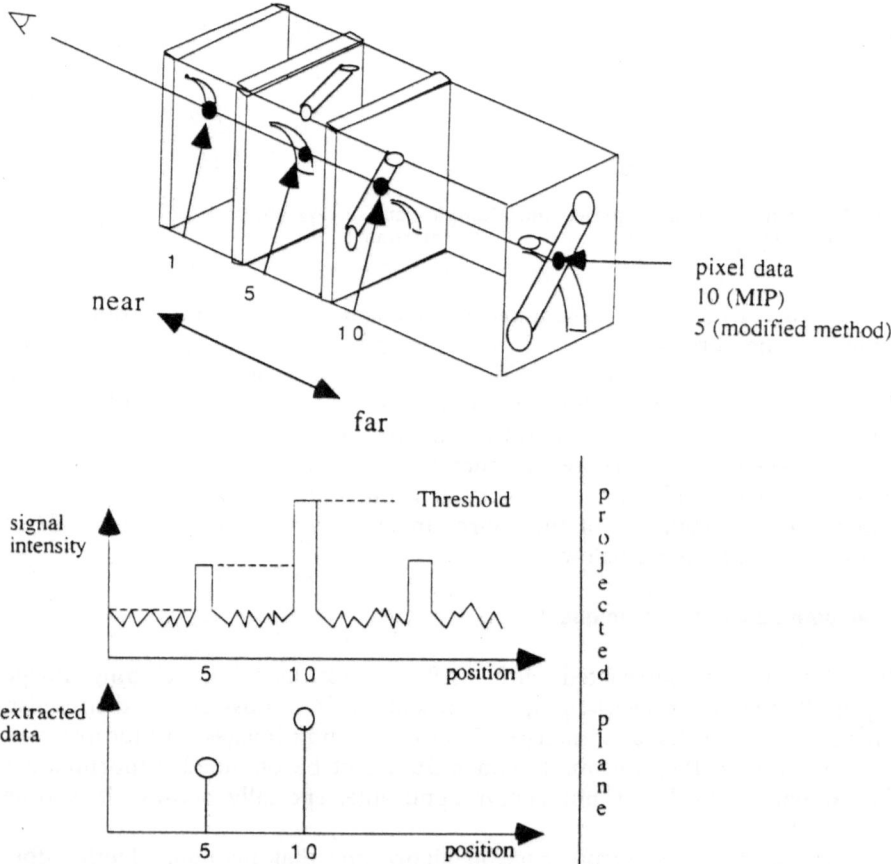

**Fig. 14.** Volume rendering technique. A different value is given to structures according to their spatial location

## Partial Volume Reformating (Targeted MIP)

With MIP, rays are projected throughout the entire imaging volume. Biliary structures are often located in a well-known area within the imaging volume. Artifacts are often present because of high signal intensity of superficial structures, especially of subcutaneous fat. Moreover, there may be artifacts caused by peristaltic motion of the duodenum, which may disturb the correct visualization of the CBD. To avoid these problems a technique called partial volume reformatting has been proposed; it is also referred to as selective MIP. The operator selects the area of interest in a limited number of slices, delineating the area in which biliary structures are present. The computer generates a MIP image, considering only the area of interest and avoiding the superficial tissues. This provides a better definition of biliary structures, especially increasing the SNR and with a better cancelation of stationary tissues.

# References

1. Patel JC, McInnes GC, Bagley JS, Needham G, Krukowski ZH (1993) The role of intravenous cholangiography in pre-operative assessment for laparoscopic cholecystectomy. Br J Radiol 66:1125–1127
2. Dawson P, Adam A, Benjamin IS (1993) Intravenous cholangiography revisited. Clin Radiol 47:223–225
3. Shehadi WH, Toniolo G (1980) Adverse reaction to contrast media. Diagn Radiol 137:299–302
4. Thomas MJ, Pellegrini CA, Way LW (1982) Usefulness of diagnostic tests for biliary obstruction. Am J Surg 114:102–108
5. Laing FC, Jeffrey RB, Wing VW, Nyberg DA (1986) Biliary dilatation: defining the level and the cause by real-time US. Radiology 160:39–42
6. Pasanen P, Partanen K, Pikkarainen P et al (1992) Ultrasonography, CT and ERCP in the diagnosis of choledocal stones. Acta Radiol 33:53–56
7. Kullman E, Borch K, Tarpila E et al (1984) Endoscopic Retrograde Cholangiopancreatography (ERCP) in patients with jaundice and suspected biliary obstruction. Acta Chir Scand 150:657–663
8. Osnes M, Myren J (1975) ERCP in patients with Bilroth II partial gastrectomy. Endoscopy 7:227–232
9. Lotveit T, Skar V, Osnes M (1988) Juxtapapillary duodenal diverticula. Endoscopy 20:175–178
10. Buset M, Dunham F, Gulbisa A et al (1991) Complications tardive de l'endoscopie diagnostique et operatoire des voies bilio-pancreatique. Acta Gastroenterol Bel 44:396–403
11. Hart R, Classen M (1990) Complications of diagnostic gastrointestinal endoscopy. Endoscopy 22:219–223
12. Lenriot J, Le Neel J, Hay J et al (1993) Cholangio-pancreatographie retrograde et sphincterotomie endoscopique pou lithiase biliare. Gastroenterol Clin Biol 17:244–250
13. Hamilton I, Lintott DJ, Rothwell J, Axon ATR (1983) Acute pancreatitis following endoscopic retrograde cholangiopancreatography. Clin Radiol 34:543–546
14. Chien D, Edelman RR (1992) Fast magnetic resonance imaging. In: Higgins CB, Hricak H, Helms CA (eds) Magnetic resonance imaging of the body. Raven, New York, pp 175–198
15. Margosian P, Schmitt F, Purdy D (1986) Faster MR imaging: imaging with half the data. Health Care Instrum 1:195–197
16. Haase A, Frahm J, Matthaei D et al (1986) FLASH imaging: rapid NMR imaging using low flip angle pulses. J Magn Reson 67:258–266
17. Haacke EM, Tkach J (1990) A review of fast imaging techniques and applications. AJR 155 (5):951–964

18. Buxton RB, Fisel CR, Chien D, Brady TJ (1989) Signal intensity in fast imaging. J Magn Reson 83 (3):576–585
19. Elster AD (1993) Gradient-echo MR imaging: techniques and acronyms. Radiology 186:1–8
20. Wehrli FW (1990) Fast-scan magnetic resonance: principles and applications. Magn Reson Q 6:165–236
21. Gyngell ML (1989) The steady-state signals in short-repetition-time sequences. J Magn Reson 81:474–483
22. Zur Y, Wood ML, Neuringer LJ (1991) Spoiling of transverse magnetization in steady-state sequences. Magn Reson Med 21:251–263
23. Cohen MS, Weisskoff RM (1991) Ultra-fast imaging. Magn Reson Imaging 9:1–37
24. Chien D, Edelman RR (1991) Ultrafast imaging using gradient echoes. Magn Reson Q 1:31–56
25. Haase A, Matthaei W, Bartkowski R, Duhmke E, Leibfritz D (1989) Inversion-recovery snapshot FLASH MR imaging. J Comput Assist Tomogr 13:1036–1039
26. Mugler JP III, Brookeman JR (1990) Three-dimensional magnetization-prepared rapid gradient-echo imaging. Magn Reson Med 15:152–157
27. Meiboom S, Gill D (1958) Modified spin-echo method for measuring nuclear relaxation times. Rev Sci Instrum 29:688–691
28. Jones KM, Mulkern RV, Schwartz RB et al (1992) Fast spin-echo imaging of the brain and spine: current concepts. AJR 158:1313–1320
29. Hennig J, Naureth A, Friedburg H (1986) RARE imaging: a fast imaging method for clinical MR. Magn Reson Med 3:823–833
30. Listerud J, Einstein S, Outwater E, Kressel HY (1992) First principles of fast spin-echo. Magn Reson Q 4:199–244
31. Nghiem HV, Herfkens RJ, Francis IR et al (1992) The pelvis: T2 weighted fast spin-echo MR imaging. Radiology 185:213–217
32. Smith RC, Constable RT, Reinhold C et al (1994) Fast Spin echo STIR imaging. J Comput Assist Tomogr 18:209–213
33. Chan TW, Listerud J, Kressel HY (1991) Combined chemical-shift and phase-selective imaging for fat-suppression: theory and clinical experience. Radiology 181:41–47
34. Axel L, Summers RM, Kressel HY, Charles C (1986) respiratory effects in two-dimensional Fourier transform MR imaging. Radiology 160:795–801
35. Wood ML, Henkelman MR (1985) MR image artifacts from periodic motion. Med Phys 12:143–151
36. Wood ML, Runge VM, Henkelman MR (1988) Overcoming motion in abdominal MR imaging. AJR 150:513–522
37. Perman WH, Moran PR, Moran RA, Bernstein MA (1986) Artifacts from pulsatile flow in MR imaging. J Comput Assist Tomogr 10:473–483
38. Ehman RL, Felmlee JP (1990) Flow artifact reduction in MRI: a review of the roles of gradient moment nulling and spatial presaturation. Magn Reson Med 14:293–307
39. Chernish SM, Maglinte DD (1990) Glucagon: common untoward reactions – review and recommendations. Radiology 177:145–146
40. Tyrell RL, Gluckert K, Pathria M, Modic MT (1988) Fast three-dimensional MR imaging of the knee: comparison with arthroscopy. Radiology 166:865–872
41. Adam G, Bohndorf K, Drobnitzky M, Guenther RW (1989) MR imaging of the knee: three-dimensional volume imaging combined with fast processing. J Comput Assist Tomogr 12 (6):984–988
42. Frahm J, Hasse A, Matthaei W (1986) rapid three-dimensional MR imaging using the FLASH technique. J Comput Assist Tomogr 10:363–368
43. Wallner BK, Schumacher KA, Weidenmaier W, Friedrich JM (1991) Dilated biliary tract: evaluation with MR cholangiography with a T2-weighted contrast-enhanced fast sequence. Radiology 181:805–808
44. Morimoto K, Shimoi M, Shirakawa T et al (1992) Biliary obstruction: evaluation with three-dimensional MR cholangiography. Radiology 183:578–580
45. Ishizaki Y, Wakayama T, Okada Y, Kobayashi T (1993) Magnetic resonance cholangiography for evaluation of obstructive jaundice. Am J Gastroenterol 88:2072–2077
46. Hall-Craggs MA, Allen CM, Owens CM et al (1993) MR cholangiography: clinical evaluation in 40 cases. Radiology 189:423–427
47. Reinhold C, Guibaud L, Genin G, Bret PM (1995) MR cholangiopancreatography: comparison between two-dimensional fast spin-echo and three-dimensional gradient-echo pulse sequences. JMRI 4:379–384

48. Outwater EK (1993) MR cholangiography with a fast spin-echo sequence. JMRI 3:131
49. Meakem TJ, Holland GA, Mc Dermott VGM et al (1993) Fast spin echo multicoil magnetic resonance cholangiography: initial experience. In: Society of Magnetic Resonance Imaging Abstract Book, p 47
50. Takehara Y, Ichijo K, Tooyama N et al (1994) Breath-hold MR cholangiopancreatography with a long-echo-train fast spin-echo sequence and a surface coil in chronic pancreatitis. Radiology 192:73–78
51. Guibaud L, Bret PM, Reinhold C, Atri M, Barkun ANG (1994) Diagnosis of choledocholithiasis: value of MR cholangiography. AJR 163:847–850
52. Shiono T, Iwasaki N (1995) MR cholangiography with fast imaging scheme. In: Society of Magnetic Resonance Imaging abstract book, p1454
53. Laubenberger J, Buchert M, Schneider B, Blum U, Hennig J, Langer M (1995) Breath-hold projection magnetic resonance cholangiopancreatography (MRCP): a new method for examination of the bile and pancreatic ducts. Magn Reson Med 33:18–23
54. Zuo C, Buff B, Wielopolski P, Clouse M (1995) MR cholangiography with fast imaging scheme. In: Society of Magnetic Resonance Imaging abstract book, p1445
55. Wielopolski P, Zuo C, Clouse M, Buff B (1995) Breath-hold 3D cholangiography using RARE and segmented echo planar imaging readouts. In: Society of Magnetic Resonance Imaging abstract book, p1448
56. Sananes JC, Bonnet M, Lecesne R et al (1995) Magnetic resonance cholangiography using HASTE sequence. Optimization and clinical evaluation in extrahepatic cholestasis. In: Society of Magnetic Resonance Imaging abstract book, p1453
57. Macaulay SE, Schulte SJ, Sekijima JH et al (1995) Evaluation of a non-breath-hold MR cholangiography technique. Radiology 196:227–232
58. Barish MA, Yucel EK, Soto JA, Chuttani R, Ferrucci JT (1995) MR cholangiopancreatography: efficacy of three-dimensional turbo spin-echo technique. AJR 165:295–300
59. Pavone P, Laghi A, Catalano C et al (1996) MR cholangiopancreatography (MRCP): technique optimization and preliminary results. Eur Radiol (in press)
60. Laghi A, Pavone P, Catalano C et al (1996) Non-breath-hold 3D MR-cholangiography at 0. 5T: technique optimization and clinical results. Presented at SMR Annual Meeting, April–May, 1995, New York
61. Brown DG, Riederer SJ (1992) Contrast-to-noise ratios in maximum intensity projection images. Magn Reson Med 23:130–139
62. Anderson CM, Saloner D, Tsuruda JS et al (1990) artifacts in maximum-intensity projection display of MR angiograms. AJR 154:623–629
63. Drebin RA, Carpenter L, Hanrahan P (1988) Volume rendering. Comput Graphics 22:65–74
64. Cline HE, Dumoulin CL, Lorensen WE et al (1991) Volume rendering and connectivity algorithms for MR angiography. Magn Reson Med 18:384–394

# CHAPTER 2

# Anatomy

## Introduction

The anatomy of the biliary and pancreatic ducts is well known (Figs. 1, 2); this chapter recalls a few basic concepts, considering particularly those anatomical structures that are identifiable on MR cholangiographic images in normal and in pathological conditions. We also evaluate the view of biliary ducts in conventional MR images, which are acquired in any case when a MR cholangiograpic study is performed.

## Main Bile Duct

The common bile duct (CBD) is defined as the choledocus and the main hepatic duct. According to the anatomy textbooks, these two parts of the biliary tree are differentiated by the confluence of the cystic duct [1–3]. The two parts present no significant anatomical and structural differences and are considered a single structure in MR cholangiography. It extends approximately 5–15 cm, with a slightly curvilinear course, having a convexity

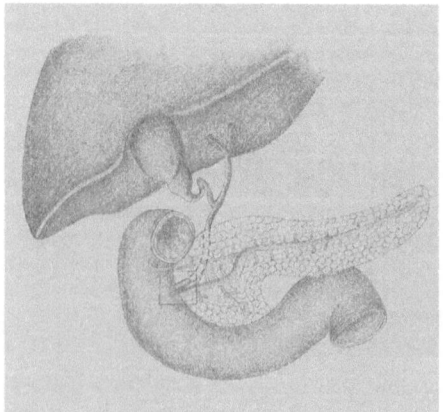
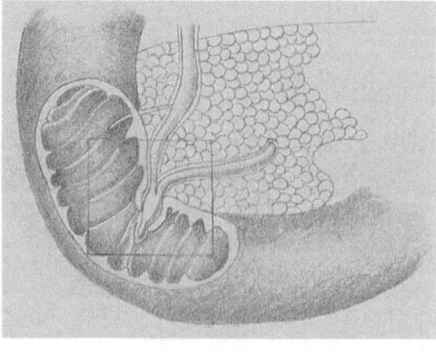

b

a

**Fig. 1. a** Diagrammatic scheme of the bile ducts showing the relationship with the surrounding organs. **b** Magnification of the region of the papilla

**Fig. 2. a** More common variants of the junction between CBD and Wirsung duct.
**b** MRCP image showing well the junction

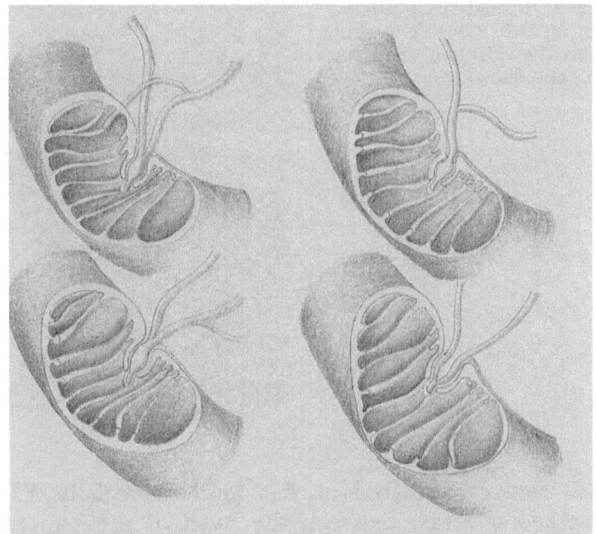

a

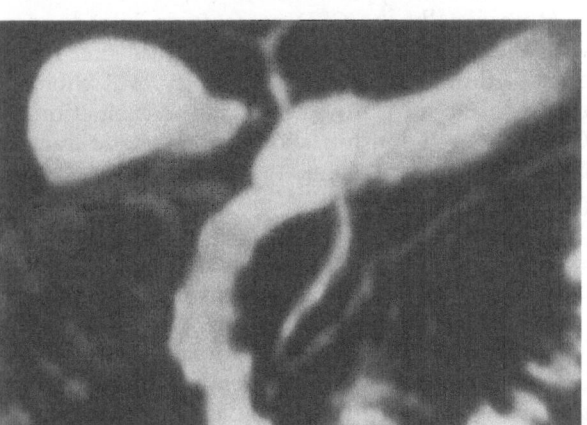

b

to the left. Its normal size is in the range of 3–10 mm; however, CBD of even 8 mm may be considered enlarged if there are symptoms (jaundice or other) [4–5].

MR cholangiography is also able to image a normal size CBD, although as a rule the larger the CBD, the stronger is the received signal and the better is the quality of the reconstructed images (Figs. 2, 3). Therefore MR cholangiography is better able to display dilated and pathological CBD than normal-sized ducts.

In the supraduodenal part the CBD is in contact with the portal vein and with the hepatic artery; immediately in a more caudal position, the main relationship is with the pancreatic head [6–7]. The type of anatomical relationship with the pancreatic head varies and is well shown in conventional axial

**Fig. 3.** Normal-sized biliary ducts. MRCP is able to show only the CBD and the main hepatic ducts

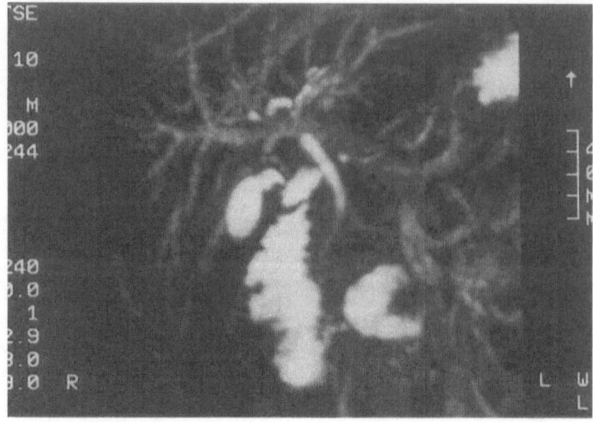

MR images acquired at this level. Especially T2-weighted images show a marked contrast between the head of the pancreas (hypointense) and the CBD (markedly hyperintense).

More distally the CBD presents an intraduodenal portion. The confluence with the pancreatic duct occurs at this site, followed by opening of the two ducts within the ampulla of Vater [8]. MR cholangiography images are sometimes not able to provide a detailed evaluation of the anatomy of the distal CBD or its relationship with the pancreatic duct and duodenum. However, by having the patient drink two cups of water prior to the examination, it is possible to obtain a fairly constant filling of the duodenum that appears hyperintense on the MR cholangiography images. In this way it is possible to determine the exact distance between the distal CBD and the duodenum to exclude the presence of masses in this area (Figs. 4–6).

As in other circumstances, the evaluation of the anatomy by means of axial conventional T2-weighted images may help the radiologist. In these images it is possible to differentiate the CBD in the intraduodenal part and the duodenal wall that surrounds it, corresponding to the papilla. With inflammatory changes in the papilla (papillitis) there is CBD dilatation without the evidence of masses in the pancreatic head or the distal bile duct. The evidence of a slightly thickened papillary wall allows the correct diagnosis of inflamatory changes of the papilla.

CBD anomalies are rare [9–10]. Duplication may occur, or an ectopic drainage in the stomach or in the third duodenal portion. The demonstration of these anomalies is theorectically possible with MR cholangiography.

## Hepatic Ducts

The two hepatic ducts are always evident in MR cholangiographic images. Usually it is possible to show the confluence and the early intrahepatic part of the hepatic ducts [11]. The left hepatic duct is usually longer and is located more anteriorly than the right hepatic duct [12]. The hepatic ducts

**Fig. 4. a** MIP-reconstructed image shows a normal-sized CBD, the cystic duct, and the gallbladder. The papilla is poorly visualized on the MIP image, but the evaluation of the source image (**b**) allows recognition of the CBD till the duodenum

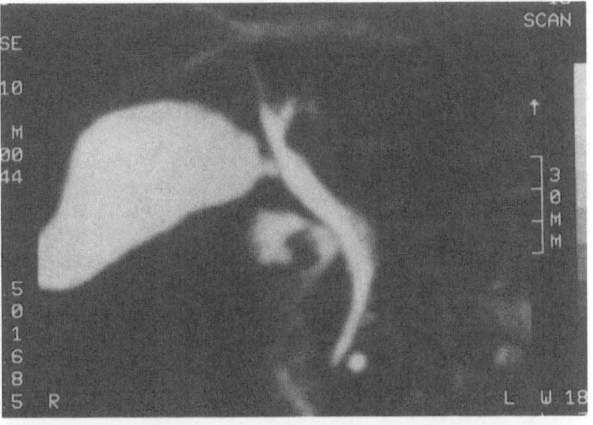

a

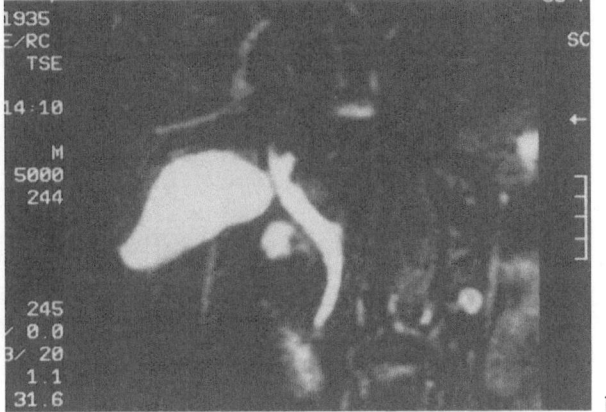

b

confluence and the first tract of the common hepatic duct are better evident in MIP-reconstructed MR cholangiography images using a right anterior oblique projection. Usually more oblique projections are evaluated to show the relative relationship of the ducts.

The intrahepatic segmental ducts are evident in MR cholangiography only with biliary ducts dilatation (Fig. 7). They are too small in normal conditions to be visualized in MR cholangiographic images. If they are evident, it is easy to display and identify anatomical anomalies, such as early drainage of the segmentary right ducts or the presence of accessory ducts draining in the right biliary ducts [13].

Conventional axial images are useful in evaluating the relationship between the hepatic ducts at the confluence, the common hepatic duct, and the portal vein. At the hepatic hilum the portal vein is localized posteriorly, with the hepatic duct in an anterolateral position, and the hepatic artery in an anteromedial position [14].

**Fig. 5. a** Correct opacification of the duodenum with
administration of tap water
is essential to demonstrate
the region of the papilla.
Also in this case the distal
tract of the CBD is not
visible on MIP image (**a**)
but only on source image (**b**)

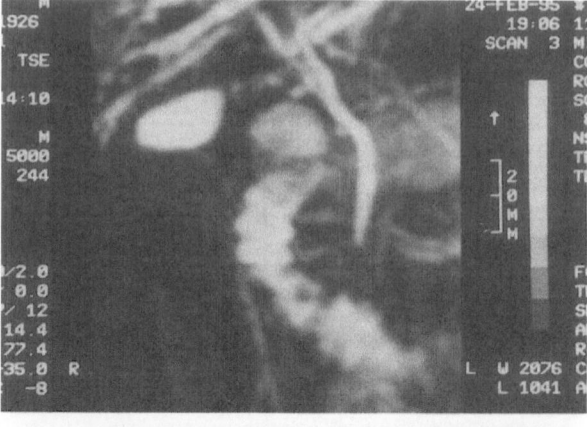

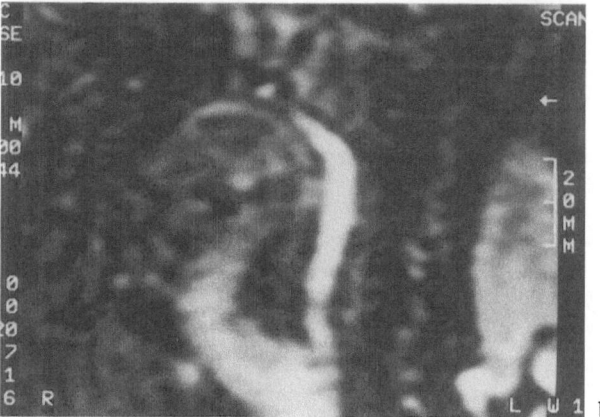

## Gallbladder and Cystic Duct

The gallbladder, more that other organs in the body, presents a very large
series of potential morphological configurations, and their description is
only indicative [15, 16]. Usually it is 8–10 cm long and 4–5 cm wide. The
size also varies according to the status of the patient, with relative ectasia in
fasting condition. Usually it is advisable to study the patient with MR cholangiography during fasting to better display the anatomy of the gallbladder.
The gallbladder is usually oriented along an oblique axis directed cranio-
caudally and from left to right. The position and course of infundibulus and
cystic duct vary depending on the location of the gallbladder.

The internal structure of the wall of the gallbladder is not evident in MR
cholangiography. Therefore we cannot determine the values for the infundi-
bulum. However, here it is possible to identify areas of absence of signal related to the presence of limited amount of bile, not evident in the MR cholangiographic images. Also, the cystic duct is not routinely evident in MR

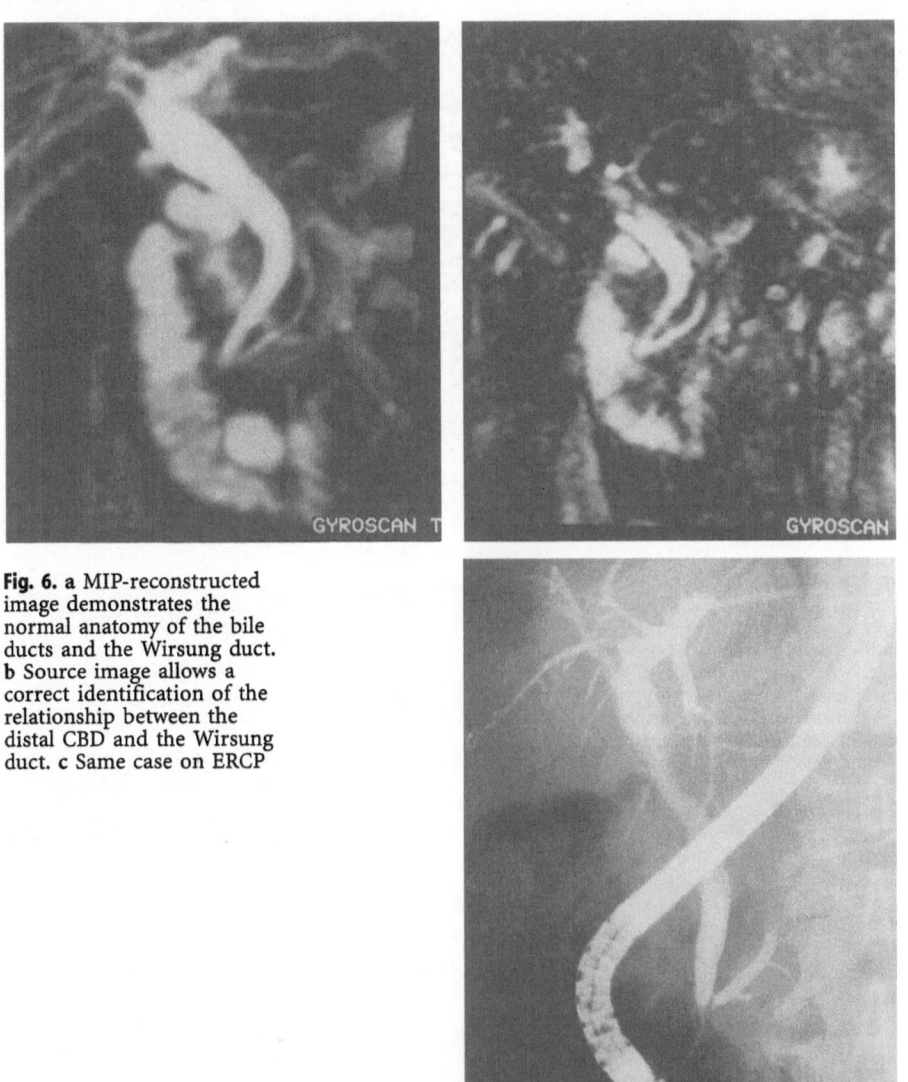

**Fig. 6. a** MIP-reconstructed image demonstrates the normal anatomy of the bile ducts and the Wirsung duct. **b** Source image allows a correct identification of the relationship between the distal CBD and the Wirsung duct. **c** Same case on ERCP

cholangiography in its complete length. Usually its evidence is improved in the distention phase of the gallbladder or in presence of a global dilatation of the biliary tree.

There are a large number of anomalies of the gallbladder, all of which are evident in MR cholangiography. These range from agenesia to complete du-plicatio. While both of these are rare anomalies, evidence is frequent of anomalies of position, with a possibly intrahepatic, transverse, or left gall-

**Fig. 7.** The two hepatic ducts are always evident on MRCP images

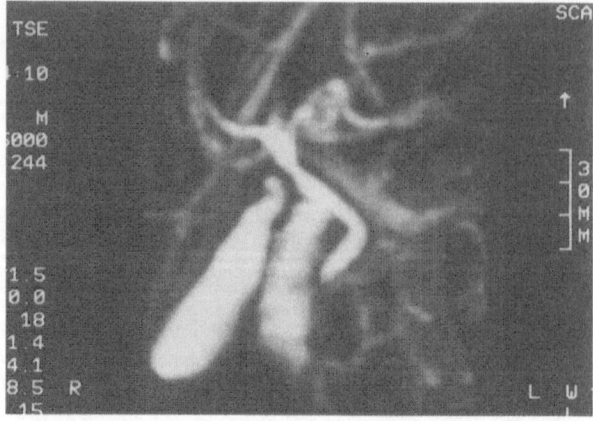

**Fig. 8. a** MIP-reconstructed image showing the CBD, the hepatic ducts, and the gall-bladder with a tortuos cystic duct. **b** An oblique projection allows the visualization of the insertion of the cystic duct on the middle porton of the CBD

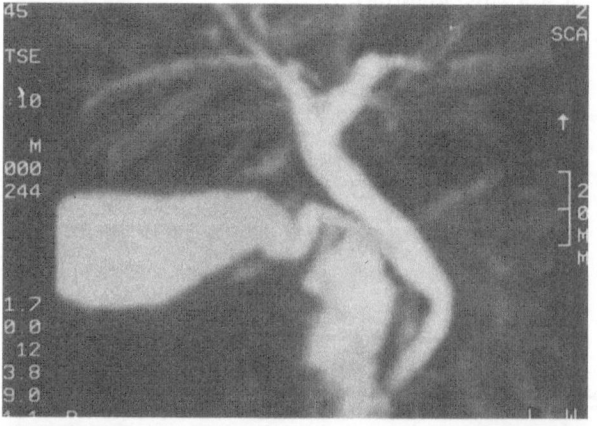

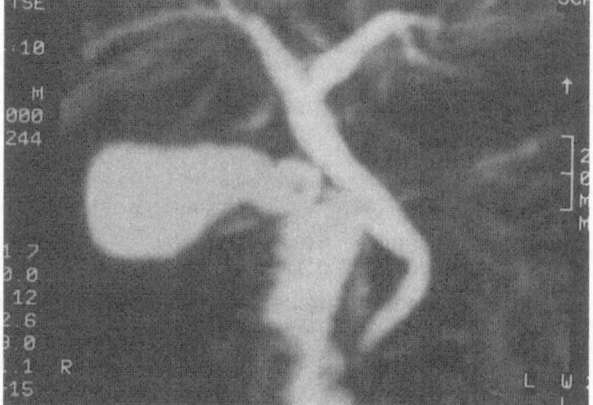

bladder, or a galbladder floating in the peritoneal cavity. More important are the anomalies of insertion of the cystic ducts because of the effect which they may have on gallbladder surgery (Fig. 8). Drainage of the cystic duct may be more cranial or more caudal than normal [16–17]. In distal drainage the cystic duct appears to be parallel to the CBD, draining just before the intraduodenal part of the choledocus. More cranial drainage can be the cause of complications during removal of the gallbladder [18].

The evidence of anomalies of the gallbladder can be achieved with MR cholangiography, particularly when high-resolution techniques are employed. Taourel et al. [19] have shown in a retrospective study that MR cholangiography can define the presence of anomalies of the drainage of the cystic duct. A prior cost–benefit analysis is necessary for the use of MR cholangiography in evaluating cystic duct anomalies or other pathologies (e.g., CBD stones) in patients to be treated by gallbladder removal [19].

## References

1. Netter FH, Oppenheimer E (1964) Liver, biliary tract and pancreas. In: The Ciba collection of medical illustrations, vol 3. Digestive system. Ciba Pharmaceutical, Summit, NJ
2. Orlof MJ (1991) The biliary system. In: Sabiston DC (ed) Textbook of surgery. Saunders, Philadelphia
3. Nahrwold DL (1991) The biliary system. In: Sabiston DC (ed) Textbook of surgery. Saunders, Philadelphia
4. Parulekar SG (1979) Ultrasound evaluation of common bile duct size. Radiology 133:703–707
5. Parke WW, Michels NA, Ghosh GM (1963) Blood supply of the common bile duct. Surg Gynecol Obstet 117:47–53
6. Boyden EA (1957) The anatomy of the choledochoduodenal junction in man. Surg Gynecol Obstet 104:641–652
7. Berland LL, Lawson TL, Foley WD (1982) Porta hepatis: sonographic discrimination of bile ducts from arteries with pulsed Doppler with new anatomic criteria. AJR 138:833–840
8. Schwartz SI (1989) Gallbladder and extrahepatic biliary system. In: Schwartz SI, Shives GT, Spencer FC (eds) Principles of surgery. McGraw-Hill, New York
9. Hayes MA, Goldenberg IS, Bishop CC (1958) The development basis for bile duct anomalies, Surg Gynecol Obstet 107:447–456
10. Jacobson JB, Brodey PA (1981) The transverse common duct, AJR 136:91–95
11. Kelvy DE, Wood RL, Enders AC (1984) Bailey's textbook of microscopic anatomy. Williams and Wilkins, Baltimore
12. Friedman AC, Sachs L (1987) Embryology, anatomy, histology and radiological anatomy. In Friedman AC (ed) Radiology of the liver, biliary tract, pancreas and spleen. Williams and Wilkins, Baltimore
13. Schulte SJ, Baron RL, Teefy SA et al (1990) CT of the extrahepatic ducts: wall thickness and contrast enhancement in normal and abnormal ducts. AJR 154:79–85
14. Michels NA (1981) Blood supply and anatomy of the upper abdominal organs with a descriptive atlas. Lippincott, Philadelphia
15. Meilstrup JW, Hopper KD, Thieme GA (1991) Imaging of gallbladder variants. AJR 157:1205–1208
16. Hollinshead WH (1971) Anatomy for surgeons, vol 2. The thorax, abdomen and pelvis. Harper and Row, New York
17. Parulekar SG (1989) Sonography of the distal cystic duct. J Ultrasound Med 8:367–373
18. Anson BJ, McVay CB (1971) Surgical anatomy, vol 1. Saunders, Philadelphia
19. Taourel P, Bred PM, Reinhold C et al (1995) MR cholangiography. Anatomic variants of the biliary tree. Radiology. 197:312

# CHAPTER 3

# Congenital Dilatation of the Biliary System

## Introduction

Congenital dilatation of the biliary ducts is a rare anomaly affecting the extrahepatic or intrahepatic biliary tree, or both. The first description of this pathological entity was that of Vater in 1723 [1], but only in the twentieth century did Vachel and Stevens (1906) and later Caroli (1958) [2] give a more detailed definition, with a classification provided by Todani in 1977 [3].

The present number of described cases in the international literature is nearly 4000, of which two-thirds are in Asia. In Oriental populations this disease affects 1 of 1000 newborns (0.01%), while in the West it affects only 1 in 100 000–150 000 newborns. Women are clearly prevalent, the female–male ratio fluctuating between 2.4:1 and 4:1 depending on the authors. The diagnosis is reached at in 50% of patients during the first decade of life and in 83% before the third decade.

The etiopathogenesis of the congenital dilatation of the biliary tree is not well known, and several theories have been put forward in recent years [5–9]. The most probable is that of Babbitt [10], who considers an anomalous insertion of the choledochus in the pancreatic duct to be responsible for the chronic reflux of the pancreatic digestive enzymes in the biliary duct. These enzymes would provoke an inflammation leading to dilatation and fibrosis. This theory is supported by demonstration of the anomalous biliary-pancreatic junction with ERCP in a proportion of cases varying between 10.5% and 58%.

## Classification

Classification of the congenital dilatation of the biliary duct is a problem. From the beginning of the century until today various authors have proposed many classifications. Based on 94 cases Alonso-Lej [11] in 1959 distinguished three different main categories. The most widely used classification is Todani's [3], based on the observations of Alonso-Lej but more developed. This classification is based on five major types (Fig. 1). The first type (80%–90% of cases) encompasses the hepatocoledochal dilatation subdivided into 1A (total cystic dilatation), 1B (segmentary cyst), and 1C (totally fusiform). Type 2 (2% of cases) is actually diverticulum of the choledochus. Type 3

**Fig. 1.** Todani's modification of Alonso-Lej's classification of congenital dilatation of bile ducts. Type 1A: cystic dilatation of the CBD. Type 1B: focal segmental CBD dilatation. Type 1C: fusiform CBD dilatation. Type 2: diverticulum in the CBD. Type 3: choledochocele involving only the intraduodenal portion of the duct. Type 4A: multiple intra and extrahepatic cysts. Type 4B: multiple extrahepatic cysts. Type 5: Caroli disease; single or multiple intrahepatic cysts

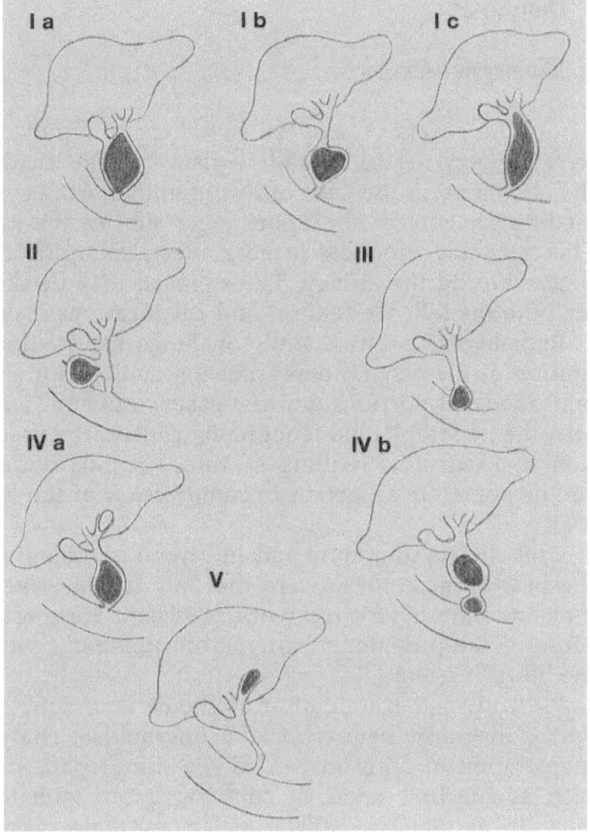

(1.4%–5% of cases) is the choledochocele in which the intraduodenal portion is dilated. Type 4 (19% of cases) includes multiple intra- and extrahepatic cystic dilatations (4A) and the extrahepatic only (4B). Lastly, type 5 is the multiple or single dilatation of the intrahepatic biliary duct, represented by Caroli disease.

## Clinical Symptoms

Clinical symptoms vary depending on the specific type of anomaly. The triad of abdominal pain, jaundice, and palpable masse is typical, although pain is the main symptom in most cases (51%) [12]. Also frequent are potential complications such as lithiasis of the gallbladder, choledocholithiasis, and the cystolithiasis, all caused by the biliary stasis present in 8%–70% of patients, and less frequently pancreatitis, ascendant colangitis, intrahepatic abscess, and biliary peritonitis caused by a spontaneous breach of the cysts. The malignant transformation is present in 2.5%–15% of the cases [13–14].

## Diagnosis

### Noninvasive Methods

Before the advent of modern radiology traditional radiological examinations were the only means for radiologists to make the diagnosis. The plain film of the abdomen, in the case of a voluminous CBD cyst, may produce a mass of medium density in the upper right side of the abdomen close to the liver. This generally produces a mass effect, enlarging the duodenal C and sometimes shifting the kidney. The stomach may be dislocated, shifted down laterally to the left. We seldom find calcifications inside the cyst [15].

Radiological contrast study of the gastrointestinal tract allows a better definition of these symptoms, showing an anterior shifting of the first and second duodenal portions and the gastric antrum. Furthermore, in choledochocele, the hypotonic duodenography can still be used, allowing the demonstration of a defect of refilling of Vater's papilla outlet. Lastly, a barium enema can demonstrate an extrinsic compression of the hepatic flexure of the colon [16].

Oral cholecystography and intravenous colangiography were often used in the past because these were the only noninvasive examinations able to demonstrate the biliary tree with precision. However, their value is limited because of the presence of a hyperbilirubinemia causing poor opacification of the biliary system [17].

Presently the examination of choice is undoubtedly echography, which allows a diagnosis before birth. Echographical study provides an accurate demonstration of both intra- and the extrahepatic dilatation. The cysts can be seen as anechoic areas in communication with them and the main biliary duct. In extrahepatic dilatation an anechoic mass can be seen next to the gallbladder, in front of the hepatic door or the pancreas head. This mass is in continuity with the biliary duct with a regular size, and no dilatation of the upstream biliary ducts can be seen. In these cases the biliary mud and gallstones are inside the cysts. In Caroli disease echography shows many intrahepatic cysts, with a consequently normal extrahepatic biliary duct. Ultrasound can also show the communication between the different cysts. This is necessary for the differential diagnosis with intrahepatic normal cysts or with multiple abscesses [18, 19].

CT may also be used to assess these anomalies, showing cystic structures with a density similar to water [20, 21]. The advantage of CT is that it can show the relationships with the surrounding structures and can be performed even in patients in whom ultrasound is disturbed by intestinal meteorism. In Caroli disease, CT can sometimes even demonstrate the communication between cysts necessary for the diagnosis. Some authors have also proposed colangiographic CT as a new method with greater accuracy than conventional CT.

## Invasive Methods

Today the gold standard for study of the congenital dilatation of the intra-
and extrahepatic biliary ducts is ERCP [22]. This method allows general vision of the biliary tree and also demonstration of the small parenchyma
branches. An accurate examination of the choledochopancreatic junction is
extremely important for defining the pathogenesis of congenital dilation of
the bile ducts. In the particular case of Caroli disease ERCP is fundamental
for the diagnosis. With the use of contrast medium it demonstrates the communication between the cystic structures. Demonstrating the communication
of these cystic structures between each other and to the biliary tree is fundamental information for the diagnosis. If the ERCP cannot be carried out due
to technical considerations, PTC can provide diagnostic images and information which are substantially the same as those obtained by ERCP. Nevertheless, each method has some limitations regarding image and technique. Image limitations are due to the fact that each shows well the structure of the
biliary ducts, but does not demonstrate other possible pathological images of
the surrounding structures. Rarely the visualization of the biliary tree can be
unsatisfactory. The technical limitations are essentially due to the invasiveness of these methods, which require interventionist maneuvers on the biliary duct (transpapillary or precutaneous approach). Each can lead to a series
of complications such as pancreatitis or cholangitis.

## Role of MRCP

The role of ERCP in the cystic dilatation of the biliary duct cannot yet be
well defined because only two studies with MRCP have been reported, one of
CBD cyst and one of Caroli disease [23, 24]. Although the casistry is miss-
ing, on the basis of personal experience and of the accuracy of the method
in the other biliary pathologies, we can presume that MRCP will in the future have a very important role in the diagnosis of this pathology. This method provides simil cholangiographic images (Fig. 2), which means images re-
presenting the biliary duct identically as the one obtained with ERCP or PTC
but without invasiveness. Considering that more than half of the cases with
congenital dilation of the bile ducts are pediatric patients or in any case very
young, the possibility of working with a completely noninvasive method
without ionizing radiation or any kind of interventionist maneuver in the
biliary ducts is a very important possibility.

Furthermore, with MRCP the extrahepatic biliary ducts are always visible
even above a stenosis that could limit the ERCP examination. Furthermore,
reconstruction with the MIP algorithm allows rotation of the image on the
coronal plan. This facilitates distinction between the superimposed images
during the AP projection. All this of course is carried out during postprocessing, which means as soon as the data are acquired, and the examination is
finished.

Particularly in Caroli disease MRCP can be extremely important and could
be proposed as the only diagnostic examination (Fig. 3). In fact, even if ultra-

**Fig. 2a–c.** Caroli disease.
a Axial T2-weighted turbo
spin echo image shows
multiple cystic dilation in
the hepatic parenchyma.
b On MIP-reconstructed
image multiple intrahepatic
cysts are well evident;
typically, the CBD is spared.
c The source image is
mandatory for a correct
evaluation of the communication with bile ducts

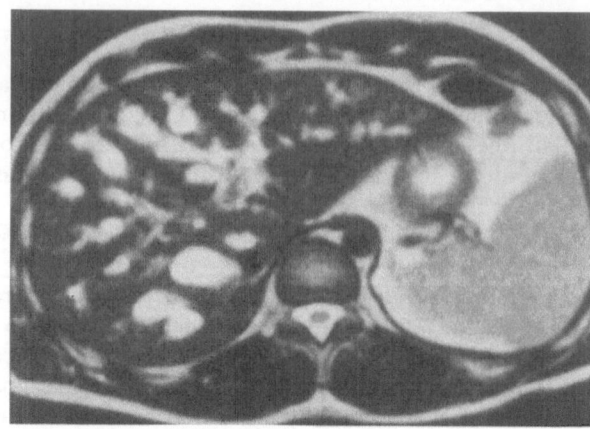

a

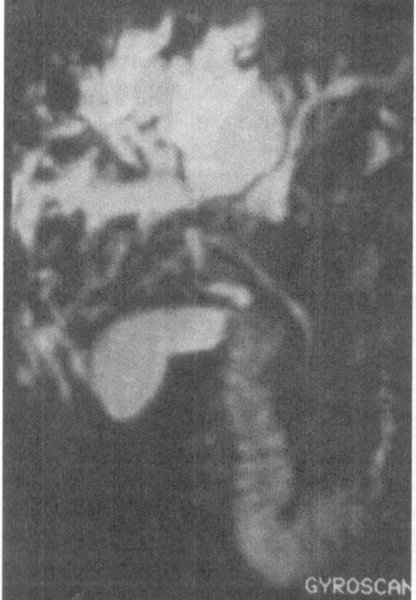

b

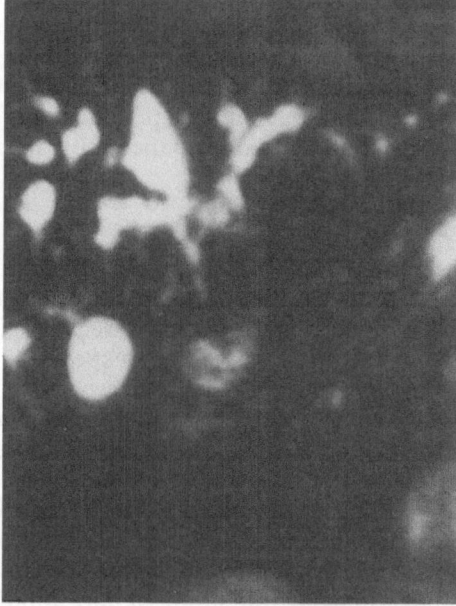

c

**Fig. 3.** Diverticulum in the CBD (type 2). MRCP MIP-reconstructed image shows the 1-cm diverticulum located in the distal part of the CBD

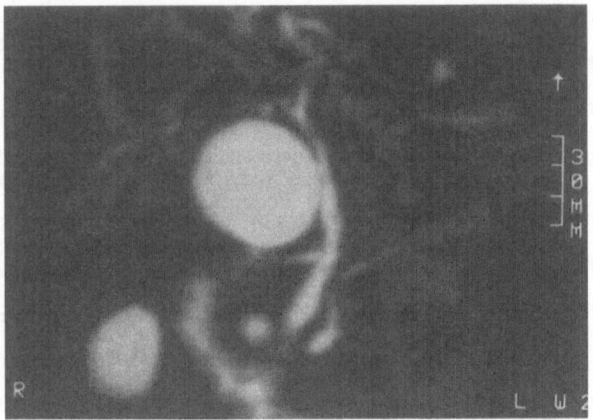

sound and CT have high accuracy in defining Caroli disease by showing multiple intrahepatic cystic structures, these methods do not always show intracystic communication or that with the biliary tree. This is a fundamental characteristic for the diagnosis. In these cases ERCP is usually performed to demonstrate the intracyst communication by using injecting contrast media inside the cysts. MRCP, with the analysis of the singular scanning, allows a simil tomographic demonstration of the very thin communications between the cysts and the biliary tree. This allows an accurate diagnosis.

## References

1. Vater A (1723) Dissertatio inauguralis medica. University Library, Edinburg, 70, II
2. Caroli J (1987) Une affection nouvelle des vpoies biliaires. La dilatation Kistique unilobaire des canaux hépatiques congénital-polykystose rénale. Proposition d'une nouvelle classification des dysembryoplasies biliaires ectasiantes de la voie biliaire principale. A propos d'unz observation. Chirurgie 113:834–843
3. Todani T, Watanabe Y, Narusue M, Tabuchi K, Kajmak C (1977) Congenital bile duct cysts. Classifications, operative procedures and review of thirty-seven cases including cancer arising from choledochal cyst. Am J Journ 134:263–269
4. Giordani M (1992) Patologia cistica intra ed extraepatica delle vie biliari. SIC 3:3–6
5. Babbitt DP, Starshak RJ, Clemett AR (1973) Choledochal cyst: a concept of etiology. Am J Roentgenol 119:57–62
6. Miyano T, Suruga K, Chen SC (1980) A clinico-pathological study of choledochal cyst. World J Surg. 4:231–238
7. Ito T, Ando H, Nagaya M, Sugito (1984) Congenital dilatation of the common bile duct in children. The etiolological significance of the narrow segment distal to the dilated common bile duct. Z Kinderchir 39:40–45
8. Wong K. C, Lister J (1981) Human fetal development of the hepatopancreatic duct junction. A possible explanation of congenital dilatation of the biliary tract. J Pediatr Surg 16:139–145
9. Kusunoki M, Yamamura T, Fujita S (1988) Choledochal cysts. Oligoganglionosis in the narrow portion of the choledochus Ann Surg 123:984–986
10. Alonso-Lej F, Rever WS, Pessagno DJ (1959) Congenital choledochal cyst, with a report of 2, and an analysis of 94 cases. Int Abstr Surg 108:1–30
11. Yamaguchi M (1980) Congenital choledochal cist. Analysis of 1433 patients in the japanese literature. Am J Surg 140:653–657

12. Tsunoda T et al (1991) Caroli's disease associated with epatolithiasis: a case report and review of the Japanese literature. Gastroenterol Jpn 26:74–79
13. Rossi RL et al (1987) Carcinomas arising in cystic conditions of the bile ducts. A clinical and pathological study. Ann Surg 205:377–384
14. Scholz F, Carrera GF, Larsen CR (1976) choledococele: correlation of radiological, clinical and pathological findings. Radiology 1118:25
15. Hess W (1987) Affezioni perinatali delle vie biliari e del pancreas. In: Hess W, Rohner A, Cirenei A, Akovbiantz A (eds) Malattie delle vie biliari e del pancreas. Fisiopatologia-Clinica-Terapia, vol 1. Piccin, Padua, p 52
16. Moreno AJ, Parker AL, Spicer MJ, Brown TJ (1984) Scintigraphic and radiographic findings in Caroli disease. Am J Gastroenterol 79:299
17. Bruneton J, Eresue J, Caramella E et al (1983) Les Kystes congenitaux du foie en echographie. J Radiology 64:471
18. Marchal GJ, Desmet VJ, Proesmans WC et al (1986) Caroli disease: high-frequency US and pathological findings. Radiology 158:507
19. Pollack M, Shirkoda A, Charnsangavej C (1985) Computed tomography of choledochocele. J Comput Assist Tomogr 9(2):360
20. Choi BI, Yeon KM, Kim SH, Han MC (1990) Caroli disease: central dot sign in CT. Radiology 174:161
21. Venu RP, Geenen JE, Hogan WJ et al (1984) Role of endoscopic retrograde cholangiopancreatography in the diagnosis and treatment of choledococele. Gastroenterology 87 (5):1144
22. Cohen SM, Bernstein JR (1981) Choledochocele presenting with jaundice. Diagnosis by percutaneous cholangiogram. Dig Dis Sci 26:667
23. Pavone P, Laghi A, Catalano C, Materia A, Basso N, Passariello R (1996) Caroli's disease evaluation with MR-cholangiography (MRCP) Abdominal Imaging 21:117–119
24. Kubo S, Kinoshita H, Higaki I, Nishio Hiroshi (1996) Choledocal cyst detected by MR cholangiopancreatography. AJR 164:513–514

# CHAPTER 4

# MR Cholangiography in Evaluation of Jaundiced Patients

## Introduction

Jaundice is a frequent clinical condition, related to the excretion or production of bile. According to the classical medical concept, still valid in the age of computerized medicine, jaundice is divided according to the cause into medical jaundice or hepatocellular jaundice, associated with a liver parenchyma alteration or dysfunction, and surgical jaundice, associated with an obstacle in the excretion of the regularly produced bile [1] As a rule, when there is no biliary tree dilatation, medical jaundice is usually considered, while if there is dilatation, stasis of bile and surgical jaundice should be considered. Exceptions to this rule include stasis conditions associated to a chronic hepatic disease (cirrhosis), in which the biliary dilatation is not present due to the impossibility of intrahepatic ducts to dilate in the nonelastic liver parenchyma.

At the first diagnostic level to face in evaluating jaundice is the distinction between the two forms. Invasive treatments (either surgical, endoscopic, or radiological) is limited to the stasis jaundice forms. Subsequently the problems related to the site and the definition of the cause of the obstructive jaundice are considered. The cause of obstructive jaundice is generally neoplastic pancreatic disease (26%–47%), CBD lithiasis (19%–42%), or other benign (e.g., papillitis, pancreatitis) or malignant causes (e.g., biliary neoplasm, hepatic hilar lymphoadenopathies) [2–4].

This chapter evaluates diagnostic findings in jaundice and the morphological aspects and possible indications to jaundice evaluation by MR cholangiography.

## Present Noninvasive Diagnostic Procedures for Evaluation of Jaundice

### Ultrasound

In present clinical practice it is easy to distinguish by ultrasound between medical and surgical jaundice as this method demonstrates biliary dilatation with very high accuracy. In the initial phases of obstructive jaundice intrahepatic biliary dilatation may not yet be present, and it is therefore necessary to study the extrahepatic biliary tree before excluding a biliary stasis [5]. The main biliary system size must to be assessed on the basis of the patient's age. A size of 5 mm is within the normal limits up to 50 years of age. Thereafter larger sizes are frequent in the absence of disease. Furthermore, in most of patients undergoing cholecystectomy a slight dilatation of the main biliary system is present [6].

Examining the intrahepatic biliary system may also help to characterize obstructive jaundice. In healthy patients the segmental intrahepatic biliary system does not exceed 2 mm in size; in the presence of dilatation the size corresponds to that of the portal branch, with the usual "gun barrel" ultrasound pattern. In addition to defining the presence of biliary dilatation, ultrasound can also assess the biliary obstruction site and cause, albeit with limited accuracy – between 27% and 95% according to different studies [7]. The variability is obviously related to the ultrasonographic experience of the operator, the patient's constitution, and the presence of meteorism.

## Computed Tomography

The role of CT is secondary to that of ultrasound, and its use is limited to cases with ascertained biliary dilatation and therefore with obstructive jaundice [8]. The major indications are noncalculous diseases. In the case of suspected lithiasis ERCP with therapeutic role is implicit.

Rapid scanning techniques and routinely injecting contrast agents during the CT examinations shows intra- and extrahepatic biliary dilatation as linear or circle hypodense structures joined with the portal branches at the intrahepatic level, at the hilum, or in the intrapancreatic site at the extrahepatic level. With the evaluation of these aspects it is possible to define the obstruction level with an accuracy over 90% [9].

To determine the cause it is necessary to evaluate both the biliary system and the surrounding structures. In a classic study, Pedrosa described the morphological aspects needed to differentiate the biliary benign obstructions from the malignant ones on CT axial scans [10, 11]. Viewing the last circle images referring to the main biliary system dilatation can help in this differentiation. The presence of irregularities of the last circle image or a sudden size reduction suggest a neoplastic lesion. On the other hand, a progressive reduction in size in the circle images, with homogeneous aspect, suggests a long segmental stenosis; this is a probable benign pattern. Even the higher density of biliary system wall, with a thickness over 5 mm, can suggest the diagnosis towards a primary biliary system lesion (cholangiocarcinoma or sclerosing cholangitis) [12]. The main information is obviously obtained from the surrounding structures, as one looks for the presence of extrinsic pathology compressing the biliary system or the extrabiliary extension of intrinsic pathology.

## Hepatobiliary Scintigraphy Mike

The information from hepatobiliary scintigraphy is particularly valuable for evaluating biliary function, which is indispensable in verifying surgical jaundice [1]. However, studies with iminodiacetic acid (IDA) have found some indications in evaluating early jaundice, in the absence of biliary dilatation, which are not yet detectable by ultrasound [13]. Usually, the indication is intrahepatic cholestasis evaluation. The most important indications are functional biliary dilatation, such as the postcholecystectomy biliary dilatation or Oddi's distony.

## MR Cholangiography

### Jaundice Definition

MR cholangiography is performed using a T2-weighted sequence which enhances the fluid signal, canceling completely the signal in the surrounding and nonfluid parenchymal tissues. The larger the amount of fluid, the higher is the signal and the larger is the SNR in the images acquired [14–15]. However, it is possible to visualize the main biliary system in the absence of dilatation (see Chap. 3), evaluating the dilated biliary system with improved image quality. It follows that MR cholangiography presents high sensitivity in jaundice definition – medical jaundice in absence of dilatation and surgical jaundice with biliary system dilatation [16, 17].

Of course, MR cholangiography use is secondary to ultrasound, which is able to screen for the presence of biliary system dilatation. In a possible diagnostic protocol concerning obstructive jaundice, MR cholangiography would always have to be performed after ultrasound in patients showing dilated biliary system. In cases of obstructive jaundice without biliary system dilatation, in the presence of evident clinical sign of biliary stasis (bilirubinemia mostly direct, alkaline phosphatase increase), it is in any case possible to perform MR cholangiography, with a good evaluation of biliary system and jaundice cause [18].

MR cholangiography can define exactly the biliary system morphology, indicating the size and relative extension of the dilatation and whether it affects both the intra- and extrahepatic system and the intrahepatic or extrahepatic systems alone. The absence of intrahepatic biliary system dilatation may be related to the presence of chronic pathology. In connection with biliary dilatation morphology is possible to evaluate the biliary occlusion site.

### Biliary Obstruction Site

Identifying the biliary obstruction site is fundamental in choosing the therapeutic approach. There is generally an endoscopic indication for the palliative treatment of jaundice in inferior (low) sites (peripancreatic), whereas in superior (high) occlusion (hilar) palliative treatment with percutaneous drainage is indicated (Fig. 1). Moreover, during the planning of surgery it is important to evaluate precisely the biliary system morphologically to define the best surgical approach and the biliary duct anastomosis.

Morphological images of the biliary system obtained by MR cholangiography can define the biliary occlusion site precisely (Fig. 2). Here MR cholangiography presents some advantages over other modalities that require direct opacification of the biliary system. First, it is possible to demonstrate the biliary occlusion site, the upstream dilatation, and in high stenosis the normal size downstream the occlusion, which is not always possible after contrast agent administration in ERCP or percutaneous cholangiography. Furthermore, it is possible at the same time to evaluate the duodenum, and if a correct filling with fluid is performed, demonstrating in low obstructions the gap between the dilated biliary system and the duodenum. In either case it is therefore possible to demonstrate correctly the occlusion of the lesions' length with important considerations for the staging of the lesions.

Another advantage is the possibility to evaluate three-dimensionally the biliary system, using the MIP technique on various projection angles. This provides a more accurate check of the occlusion site because it is possible to image the biliary carrefour better or to separate the distal CBD from the Wirsung and the duodenum in cases of occlusions at the papillar level [15].

**Fig. 1. a, b** T1-weighted axial scans show dilation of the intrahepatic ducts and a hypointense at the level of the hilum, causing the obstruction. **c** MRCP image demonstrates the hilar obstruction at the level of the carrefour with separation between right and left ducts. **d** ERCP confirms MRCP findings

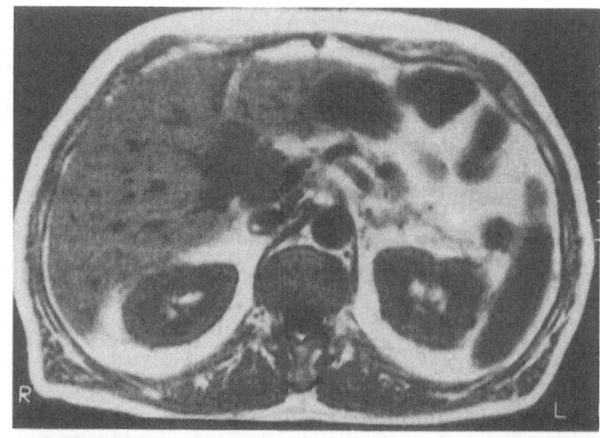

a

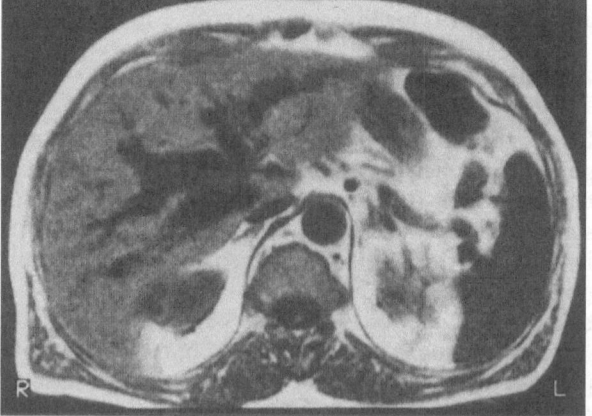

b

**Fig. 1.** (cont.)

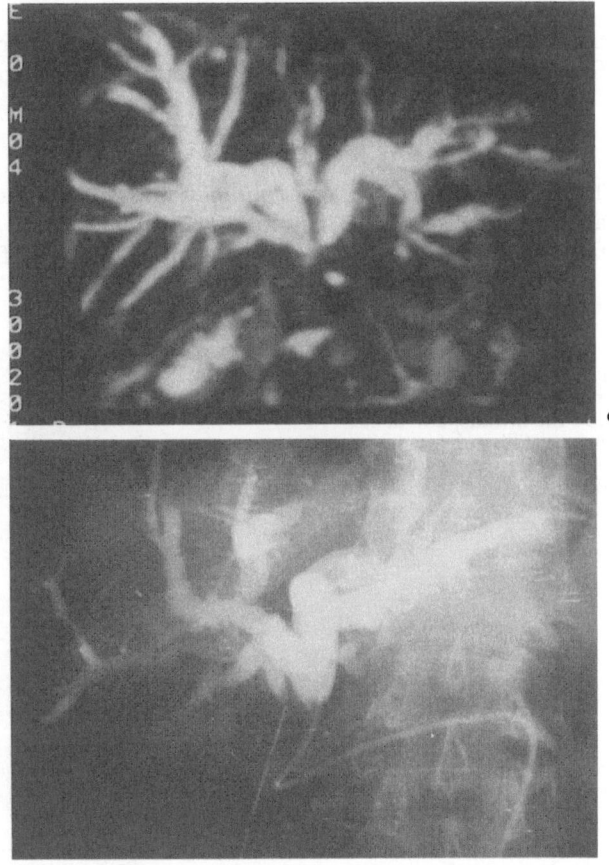

c

d

**Fig. 2.** MRCP allows recognition of the level of the obstruction in a patient with biliodigestive anastomosis (hepatico-jejunostomy)

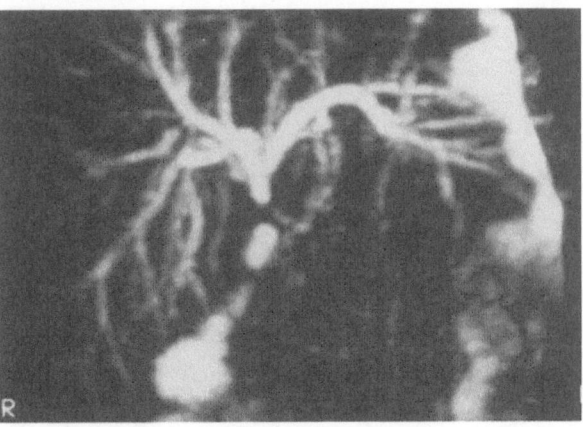

We routinely perform multiple MIP projections, with 5° from each other until they form a 180° arc. The biliary occlusion site provides important information about the cause of the occlusion (see below).

## Cause of the Obstruction

The biliary obstruction morphology and site provide important information about the cause of the jaundice. The semeiotics of the MR cholangiographic pattern in the biliary occlusion is similar to that of modalities with the bili-

**Fig. 3. a** MRCP MIP-reconstructed image demonstrates a wide dilation of the CBD and the intrahepatic ducts. A large filling defect is evident at the level of the distal CBD. **b** The source image offers a well depiction of the multiple stones inside the CBD

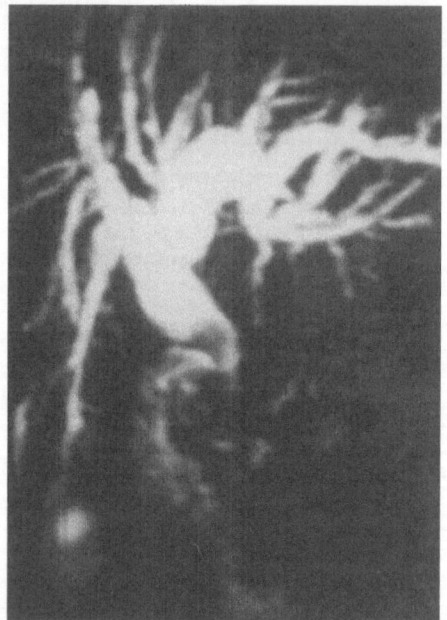

a

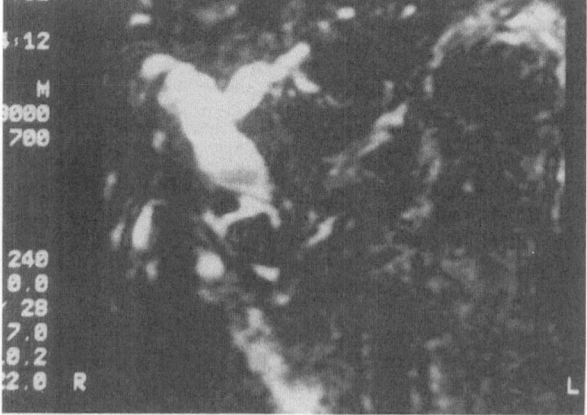

b

ary system direct opacification (ERCP, percutaneous and intraoperatory cholangiography). Although MR cholangiography generally has enough spatial resolution to evaluate the biliary system, it does not provide anatomical details identical to those of the radiological cholangiographies. Therefore subtle findings, such as those of biliary surface irregularities, cannot be detected in the same way. However, it is possible to indicate in a general way the biliary system morphology in connection with the obstructive jaundice cause.

Occlusions due to stones appear as a "concave lens" pattern of the distal part of the dilated biliary system. The stone does not present a detectable signal and thus behaves as the radiotransparent stones in the radiological examinations (Fig. 3). Occlusions due to benign stenosis present an elongated morphology of the distal biliary duct, with a lumen progressive thinning (Fig. 4). Occlusions due to neoplastic lesions present a sudden interruption of the dilated biliary duct, with distal irregular marginal aspect or with a sudden thinning aspect (Figs. 5, 6). These differential diagnostic considerations are general and not very specific and can be improved with evaluation

**Fig. 4. a** Focal mass at the level of the head of the pancreas, mimicking a pancreatic carcinoma. **b** MRCP image shows an elongated morphology of the distal biliary duct with a progressive thinning of the lumen. **c** the source image shows multiple stones in the gallbladder

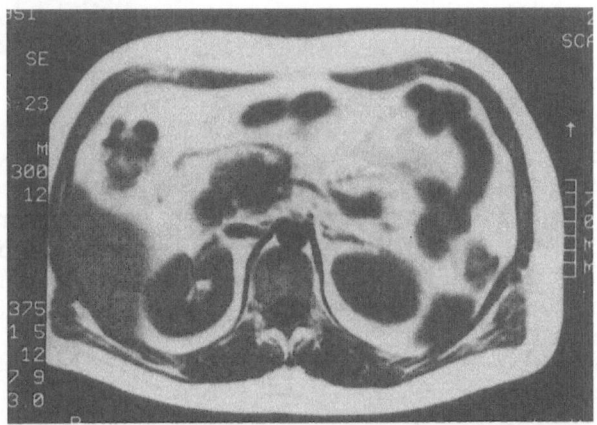

a

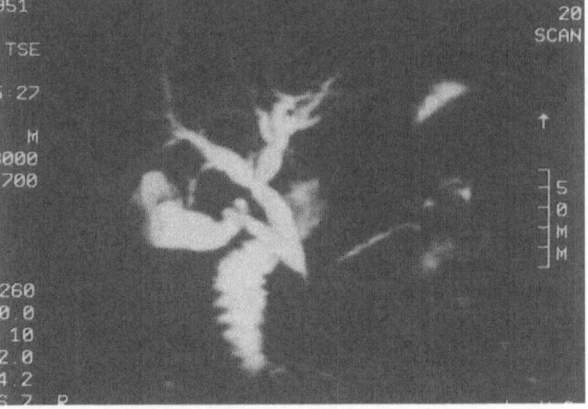

b

**Fig. 4.** (cont.)

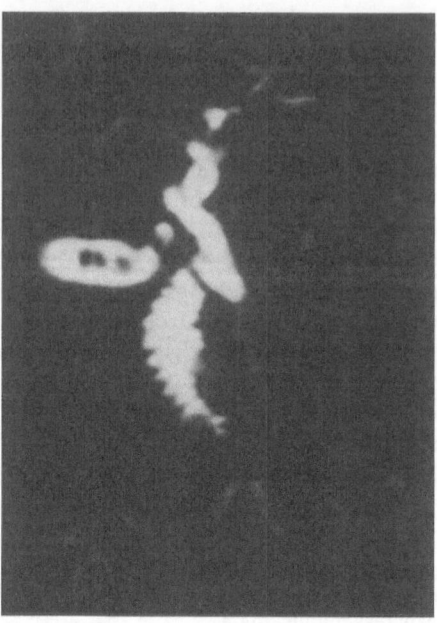

c

of the MR images always obtained in conjunction with MR cholangiographic images.

MR cholangiography is obtained by a maximum intensity projection (MIP) of single 3D sections; therefore it is always necessary to evaluate both the projection images and the single sections to identify the biliary morphology at the occlusion level or the possible filling defects not detectable on projection images. Single images are indispensable, particularly in evaluating stones.

**Fig. 5.** Carcinoma of the head of the pancreas. a Axial T1-weighted image shows a hypointense mass at the level of the head of the pancreas. b On MRCP image a sudden interruption of both the CBD and the Wirsung duct is evident

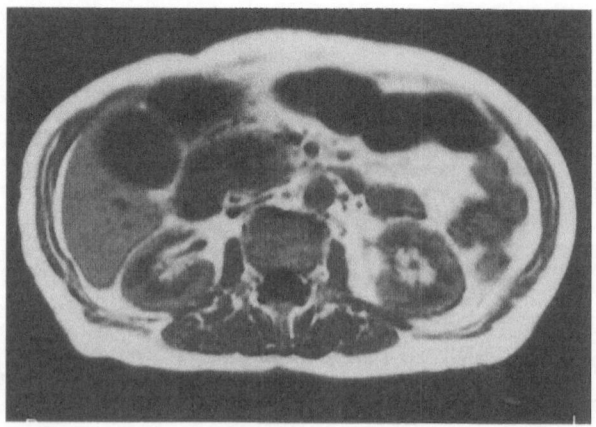

a

**Fig. 5.** (cont.)

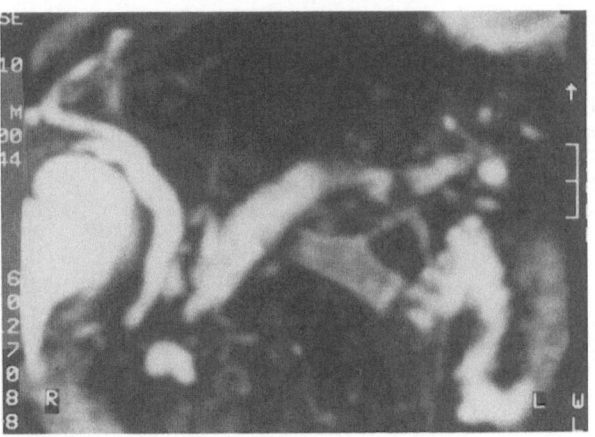

b

During MR cholangiography, MR conventional images are also obtained, which can demonstrate the surrounding anatomic structures. In addition to the indirect morphological sign of biliary involvement in pancreatic parenchymal disease or other neoplasms, it is thus possible to demonstrate directly the lesion causing the biliary involvement, with important considerations both on staging of lesions and cause definition [19].

The considerations relative to the specific causes of obstructive jaundice are discussed in the appropriate chapters.

## Role of MR Cholangiography

MR cholangiography can assume a very important role in the definition of obstructive jaundice [20]. Until now, after ultrasound, ERCP is performed with diagnostic and therapeutic aims, or CT is performed to stage the neoplastic lesions. MR cholangiography can totally replace the diagnostic role of ERCP. At the same time, it is able to provide information about lesions extension, replacing CT in neoplasm staging. Thus ERCP would find indications only in the presence of stones, with therapeutic aims, and in the advanced neoplasms, which are not resectable, to perform palliative biliary drainage (otherwise performable in transhepatic way).

In cost–benefit analyses MR cholangiography appears a valuable technique since it obviates unnecessary CT and palliative ERCP. It is routine to combine diagnostic ERCP with jaundice drainage even in operable patients. The screening offered by MR cholangiography distinguishes clearly between operable lesions and lesions which require a palliative treatment, with a better preoperative selection performed in a noninvasive way. This chapter therefore concludes with a proposal for an obstructive jaundice diagnostic protocol, such as is routinely performed in our department. Performance of MR cholangiography immediately after screening with ultrasound provides the basis for determining not only the subsequent diagnostic protocol but also

**Fig. 6.** MRCP (a) and ERCP (b) findings may mimic a pancreatic carcinoma due to the sudden interruption of both the CBD and the Wirsung duct. At surgery the mass was diagnosed as chronic pancreatitis

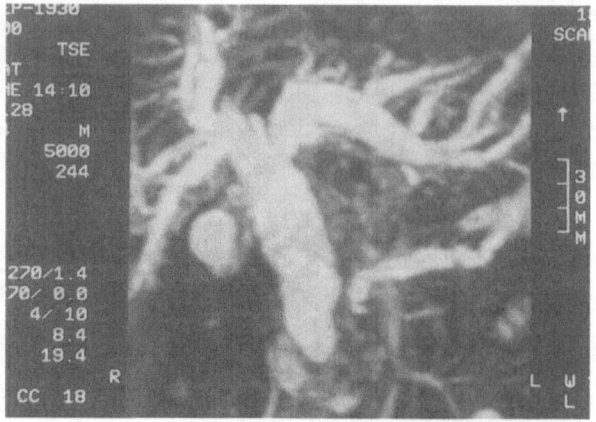

a

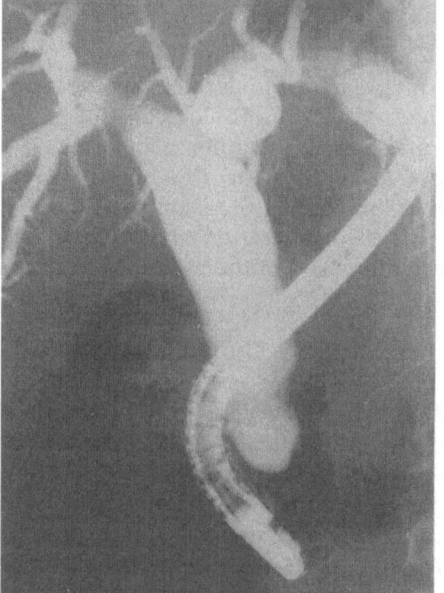

b

the therapy to be performed in individual cases, whether surgical or interventional (ERCP or radiological drainage).

## References

1. Krishnamurthy GT, Lieberman DA, Brar HS (1985) Detection, localization and quantitation of a degree of common bile duct obstruction by scintigraphy. J Nucl Med 26:726–735
2. Malchow Moller A, Thomsen C, Matzen P, Mindeholm L, Bjerregaard B, Bryant S, Hilden J, Holst-Christensen J, Johansen ST, Juhl E (1986) Computer diagnosis in jaundice. Bayes' rule founded on 1002 consecutive cases. J Hepatol 3 (2):154–163

3. Saint-Marc Girardin MF Le Minor M, Alperovitch A, Roudot-Thoraval F, Metreau JM, Dhumeaux D (1985) Computer-aided selection of diagnostic test in jaundiced patients. Gut Sept 26:961–967
4. Cronan JJ, Mueller PR, Simeone JF et al (1983) Prospective diagnosis of choledocholithiasis. Radiology 146:467–469
5. Laing FC, Jeffrey RB Jr (1983) Choledocholhitiasis and cystic duct obstruction: difficult ultrasonographic diagnosis. Radiology 146:475–479
6. Einstein DM, Lapin SA, Ralls PW et al (1984) Tha intensitivity of sonography in the detection of choledocholithiasis. AJR 142:725–728
7. Honickmann Sp, Mueller Pr, Wittenberg J et all (1983) Ultrasound in obstruction jaundice: prospective evaluation and cause. Radiology 147:511–515
8. Baron RL, Stanley RJ, Lee JKT et al (1982) A prospective comparison of the evaluation of biliary obstruction using computed tomography and ultrasonography. Radiology 145:91–98
9. Jeffrey RB Jr, Federele MP, Laing FC et al (1983) Computed tomography of choledocholithiasis. AJR 140:1179–1183
10. Pedrosa CS, Casanova R, Rodriquez R (1981) Computed tomography in obstructive jaundice. I. The level of obstruction. Radiology 139:627–634
11. Pedrosa CS, Casanova R, Rodriquez R (1981) Computed tomography in obstructive jundice II. Radiology 139:635–645
12. Schulte ST, Baron RL, Teefey SD et al (1990) CT of the extrahepatic bile ducts: wall thickness and contrast enhancement in normal and abnormal ducts. AJR 154:79–85
13. Beinart C, Stravos E, Cohen B et al (1981) Obstruction without dilatation. JAMA 245:353–356
14. Wallner BK, Schumacher KA, Weidenmaier W, Friedrich JM (1991) Dilated biliary tract: evaluation with MR cholangiography with a T2-weighted contrast-enhanced fast sequence. Radiology 181:805–808
15. Morimoto K, Shimoi M, Shirakaw T et al (1992) Biliary obstruction: evaluation with three-dimensional MR cholangiography. Radiology 183:578–580
16. Gupta RK, Kakar AK, Jena A et al (1989) Magnetic resonance in obstructive jaundice. Aust Radiol 33:245–251
17. Ishizaki Y, Wakayama T, Okada Y, Kobayashi T (1993) Magnetic resonance cholangiography for evaluation of obstruction jaundice. Am J Gastroenterol 88 (12):2072–2077
18. Hall-Craggs MA, Allen CM, Owens CM, Theis BA, Donald JJ, Paley M, Wilkinson ID, Chong WK, Hatfield AR, Lees WR et al (1983) MR cholangiography: clinical evaluation in 40 cases. Radiology 189 (2):423–427
19. Dillon E, Peel AL, Perkin GJ (1981) The diagnosis of primary bile duct carcinoma (cholangiocarcinoma) in the jaundiced patient. Clin Radiol 132:311
20. Gupta RK, Kakar AK, Jena A et al (1989) Magnetic resonance in obstructive jaundice. Aust Radiol 33:245–251

# CHAPTER 5

# Biliary Stone Detection by MR Cholangiography

## Choledocholithiasis

Common bile duct (CBD) stones are present in 6%–12% of patients with gallbladder stones who undergo cholecystectomy. Autopsy series show 4%. In these cases the stones typically migrate through the cystic duct into the CBD [1]. Once a stone is present in the CBD, each stone can increase in size or number due to the presence of biliary stasis and inflammation, always present in case of choledocholithiasis. The stones may be unique or multiple, and they can reach every tract of the CBD. However, stones can easily be stopped at the level of papilla due to the typical course and shape of the CBD, narrower in the distal tract. The clinical symptoms, when present, are quite typical: biliary colic, fever, and jaundice. Jaundice is usually intermittent or continuous, with periods of remission, usually without worsening of the symptoms; however, the patient's condition may worsen in cases of overlapping pancreatitis or cholangitis [2].

### Noninvasive Diagnostic Procedures

The noninvasive diagnosis of the choledocholithiasis presents several limitations that are related to its low sensitivity. The plain abdominal film has a limited diagnostic role, with evidence of only radiopaque stones, projecting along the course of the biliary tree.

Limited results are also obtained with intravenous cholangiography. Its greater limitation is the opacification of the biliary tract in only 30%–40% of cases. In a prospective study, intravenous cholangiography proved useful in the diagnosis of choledocholithiasis in only 1.5% of cases [3]. For this reason and due to the risks related to hypersensitivity of contrast media, the costs, the time required for completing the procedure execution, and the limited anatomical detail of the biliary tree, this procedure is not longer used [4]. Also, manufacturers have ceased the production and distribution of contrast media for intravenous cholangiography due to the high production costs and drastic reduction in the market.

The accuracy of ultrasound varies from 20% to 80%, depending on patient cooperation, operator ability, and difficulty in showing stones in a nondilated biliary tree; furthermore abdominal meteorism can limit visualization of the distal tract of the CBD. The sensitivity of ultrasound is 59%, but if the CBD is less than 6 mm, it cannot show the calculi in up to 86% of patients [5]. False positives due to the presence of hyperechoic structures such as surgical clips, endoprosthesis, and cystic duct tortuosity can occur, with reduction in diagnostic accuracy. However, the first diagnostic step in patients with clinically suspected bile duct calculi is ultrasound, due to the wide availability of the equipment and the low cost of the procedure.

CT has an accuracy comparable to that of ultrasound (23%–85%); however, it uses ionizing radiation and entails higher costs [6]. Specificity is very high with both techniques – 97% for ultrasound and 98% for CT. More recently, new studies have again established the criteria for CT diagnosis, finding low value of sensitivity (75%) [7–8]. On the whole, the noninvasive diagnosis of bile duct stones with a diagnostic accuracy of 50%–60% should not be considered adequate.

## Invasive Procedures

ERCP is often required, both for therapeutic and diagnostic purposes, especially when ultrasound does not provide consistent diagnostic information. However ERCP should be restricted to selected patients, because it is an invasive procedure and is not well tolerated by the patient, with morbidity of 10% and mortality of 0.37%–1% [9]. If we consider that the majority of patients with symptoms compatible with the presence of stones do not in fact have any, we realize how often an invasive procedure as ERCP is performed only for pure diagnostic reasons.

In selected postsurgical patients ERCP cannot be performed (e.g., hepatic or choledocho-jejunostomy), and it is difficult to perform in patients who have undergone Billroth II gastric resection or in presence of bulky retroperitoneal neoplasm, duodenal diverticuli, ampulla edema or necrosis, and ampullomi [10]. The successful rate of ERCP is 95%, but pancreatitis and cholangitis can complicate this procedure. After injecting the contrast media, the amylase level increases in 70% of patients, while pancreatitis occurs in 1% of cases. Cholangitis is seen in 4%–10% of cases, but the incidence decreases to 1% when a nasogastric drainage is inserted after the procedure. The high accuracy of ERCP in defining the cause of obstruction is well known; however, often for technical reason the overall results are somewhat limited, and a sensitivity of 76% is reported for this technque [5].

Another invasive procedure for visualizing the biliary tree is intraoperative cholangiography, currently performed during laparoscopic cholecystectomy. Not all authors agree with its value. Some consider this procedure, when performed with laparoscopy, inconvenient because it is time consuming, and because of the risks of iatrogenic damage to the CBD [11]. Its value is not questioned when the removal of CBD stones is performed with the same surgical approach; however, there is no agreement on this approach.

The last invasive procedure for the detection of CBD stones is laparoscopic ultrasound (performed during laparoscopic cholecystectomy); only limited, preliminary clinical data are available on this, and there is no evidence that it could replace intraoperative cholangiography in the future.

## MRCP

MRCP is an alternative noninvasive procedure in the study of choledocho-lithiasis [12]. The high-resolution contrast obtained in MRCP allows a clear distinction between stones and bile contained in the ducts.

### Stone Diagnosis

Independently of the calcium content, which is typically hypointense in MRI because of the lack of free protons, biliary stones always show low signal intensity in contrast to the high signal intensity of the bile (Fig. 1). In vitro studies have shown that there are limited exceptions to this rule, with evidence of streaks of higher signal intensity on stones with internal structural discontinuity, where bile can infiltrate.

MRCP is based on three-dimensional (3D) reconstruction of the images obtained by a maximum intensity projection (MIP) algorithm that provides a cholangiogram similar to that obtained by intravenous, percutaneous, or en-

**Fig. 1. a** MIP-reconstructed image shows inhomogeneous signal intensity in the distal third of the CBD without a clear evidence of a stone. **b** The source image better depicts the presence of a 9-mm stone

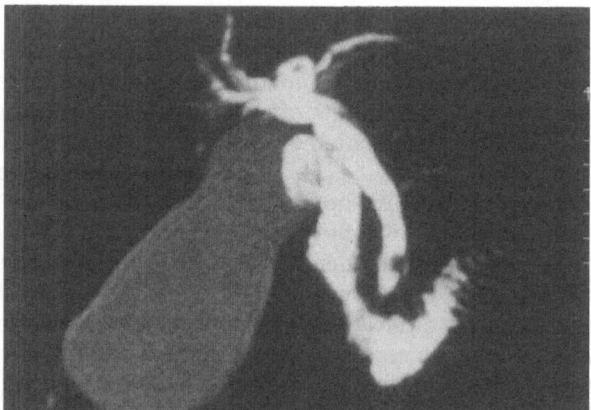

a

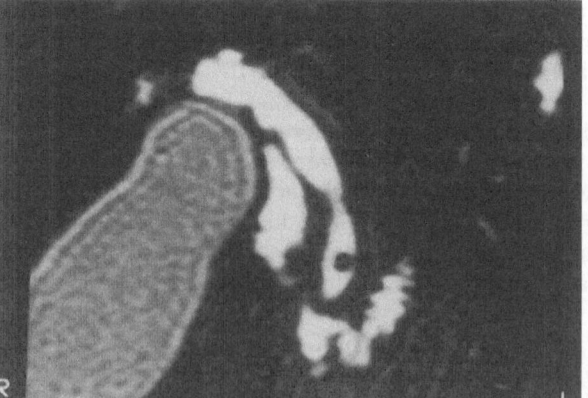

b

**Fig. 2. a** On MIP-reconstructed image a dilated CBD is observed, with evidence of a distal obstruction, but without intraluminal filling defects. **b** The source image allows the depiction of multiple stones. **c** ERCP, performed with a therapeutic purpose, confirms MRCP findings

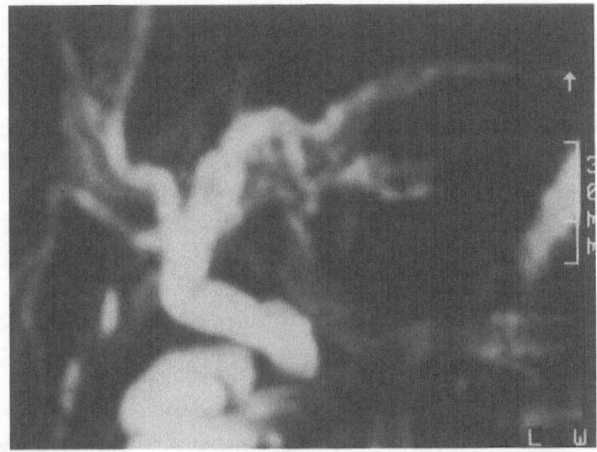

a

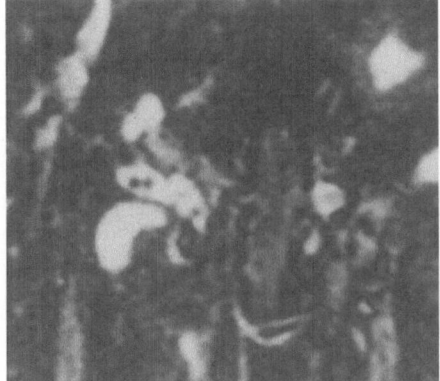

b

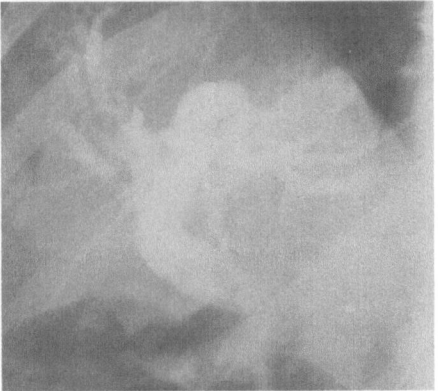

c

doscopical cholangiography so that the semeiotic features are the same [13]. Therefore the stone is depicted as a "filling defect," round or ovalar, within the CBD, which is dilated and present high signal intensity [14] (Figs. 2, 3).

When the stone is wedged in the papilla, the CBD is of low signal intensity in the distal tract, with a convex shape ("meniscus"; Fig. 4). There are no problems in depicting stones of larger size (more than 1 cm diameter). Even with the MIP reconstruction we can recognize the filling defect (Figs. 5, 6). However, to recognize the small calculi we need to evaluate the single slice acquired in the coronal plane. This type of study ("tomographic-like") is necessary in all cases because in MIP reconstruction stones can be obscured by the surrounding high signal intensity of the bile (Figs. 7, 8). The same problem can occur in the ERCP, while the high concentration of the contrast media prevents the stone visualization and localization.

**Fig. 3. a** MIP-reconstructed image showing slight dilation of the CBD, without evidence of intraluminal filling defects. **b** The 1-cm stone is well evident on the source image. **c** Also on the axial T2-weighted image the stone can be recognized

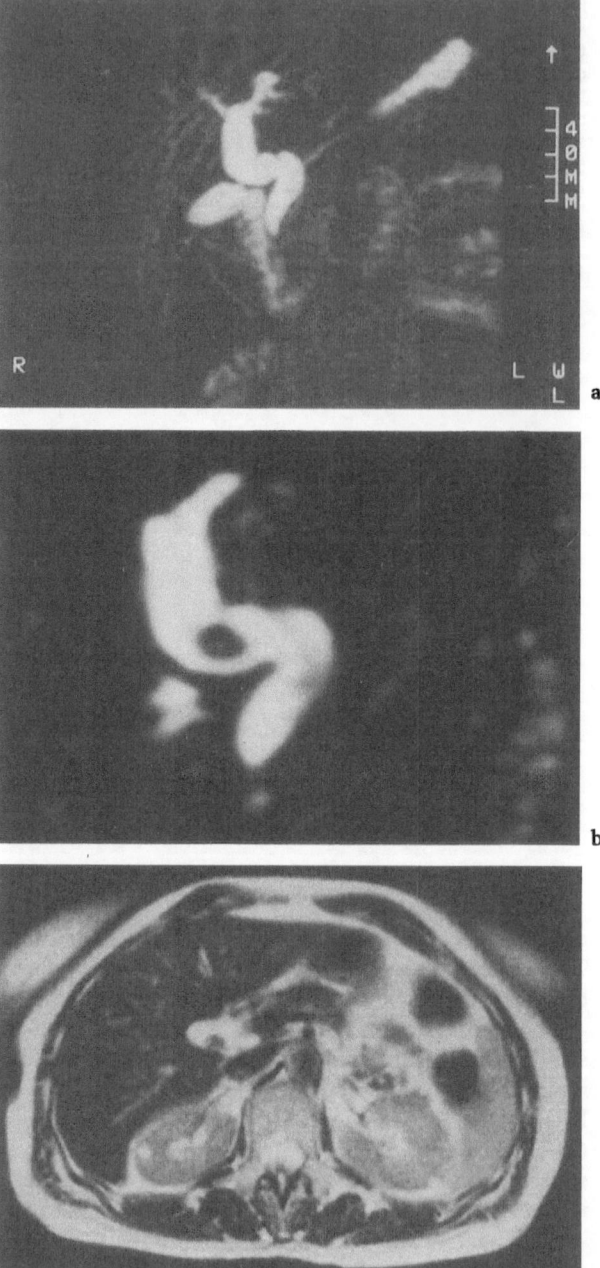

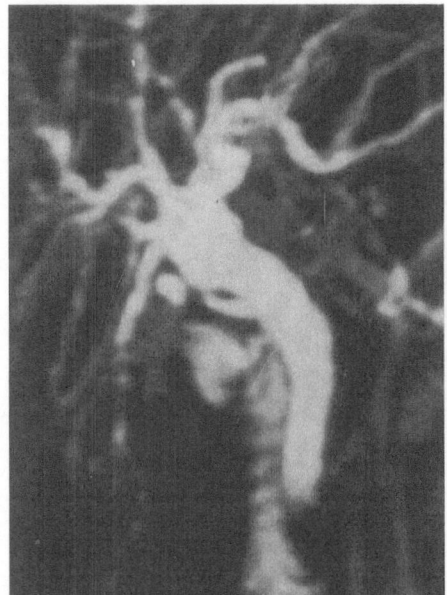

a

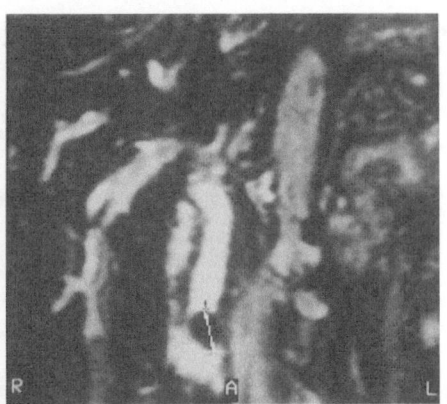

b

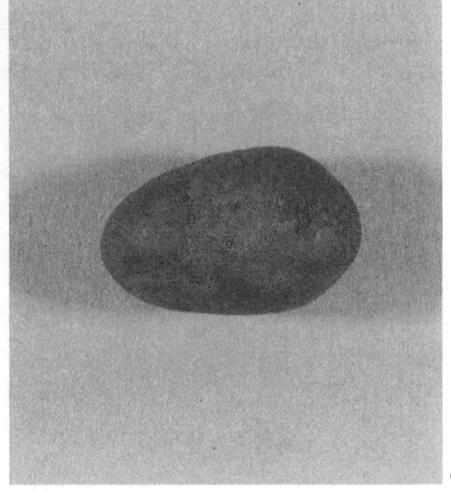

d

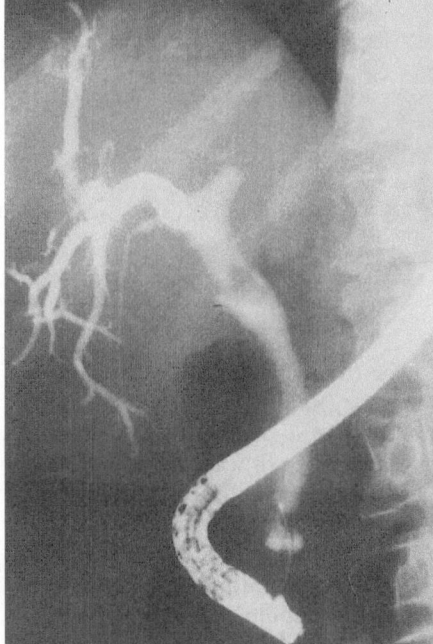

c

**Fig. 4. a** MIP-reconstructed image showing a wide dilation of the CBD and the main intrahepatic ducts secondary to a distal obstruction; a filling defects with a "meniscus sign" is appreciable. **b** On source image the 2-cm stone wedged in the papilla is evident. **c** On ERCP the stone is removed by a Dormia catheter. **d** Image of the extracted stone. **e–f** Also on the axial T2-weighted images the stone could be appreciated: on a cranial scan the high signal intensity of the CBD is well depicted (**e**), while on a caudal scan (**f**) the high signal intensity is replaced by the low signal intensity of the stone

**Fig. 4.** (cont.)

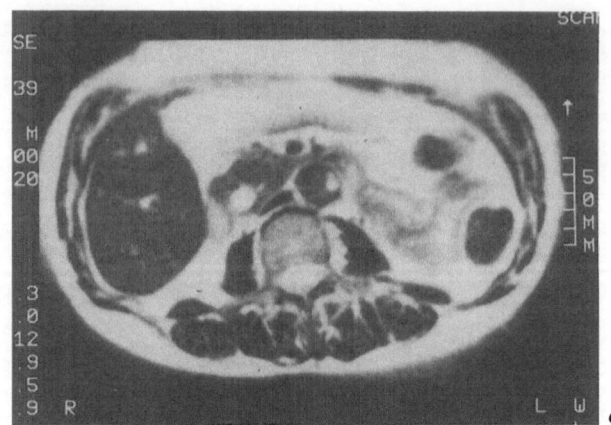

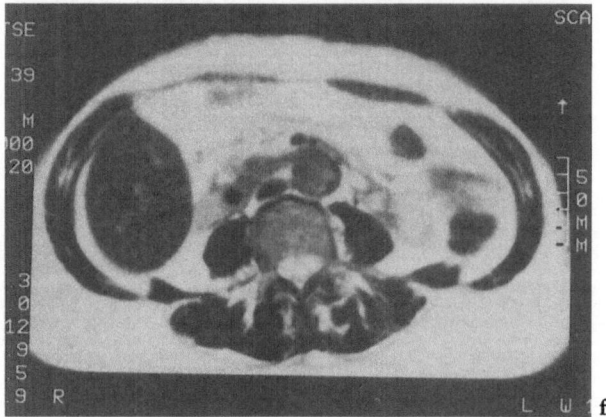

## Resolution of MRCP

Although MRCP has a spatial resolution lower than that of X-ray cholangiography with direct injection of contrast agents (namely ERCP), its higher
contrast resolution allows detection of stones up to 2–3 mm in diameter. In
our own series we had a positive MRCP in a patient with a stone of 5 mm in
diameter placed in the distal tract of the CBD, when the subsequent ERCP result was negative (Fig. 9) [15]. However, the following sphincterotomy and
baloon catheter positioning led to removal of the stone.

By MRCP we can detect multiple calculi. This technique is particularly
helpful when the presence of wedged stones in the papilla does not allow the
progresion of contrast media. Another advantage of MRCP is that we can
postprocess the images. With this technique we reconstruct the images after
the acquisition of patient data and then rotate them in multiple projections
rather than in a single projection as in ERCP [16]. In this way the stone's location can be better defined in the CBD. By rotating the image after MIP re-

**Fig. 5. a** The stone at the level of the carrefour is visible
even on MIP-reconstructed
image. **b** On the source image the 2-cm stone is clearer

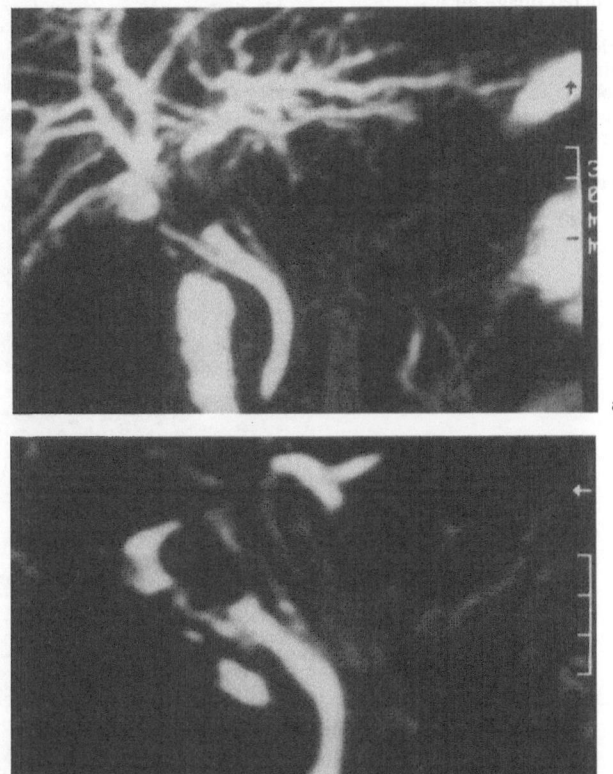

construction we are able to identify stones that are obscured in the antero-
posterior view by other anatomical structures.

### Limitations

Technical problems still lead to some limitations in currently employed procedures, but it is highly probable that in the near future these problems will
be resolved. For example, it is hard to detect small stones in the peripheral
biliary duct even if we evaluate the single coronal planes. Therefore we cannot diagnose calculi when they are small and located in the peripheral, normal-sized ducts. If the ducts are dilated, there is no problem in identifying
small stones, even in the intrahepatic ducts. Multiple stones in the CBD may
cause an inhomogeneous signal with poor depiction of the CBD (Fig. 10).
Another problem is air, which causes susceptibility artifacts; in one of our
patients with a large amount of air inside the CBD a small stone was missed
(Fig. 11).

**Fig. 6. a** On MIP-reconstructed image an in-
homogeneous signal is
evident in the middle
third of the CBD. **b** The
stone is clearly depicted
on source image. **c** The
contrast study performed
by a cholecystostomy con-
firms the presence of the
stone

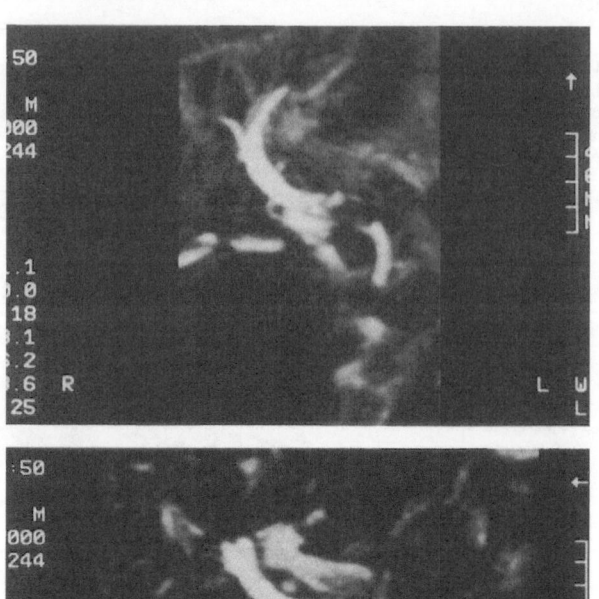

a

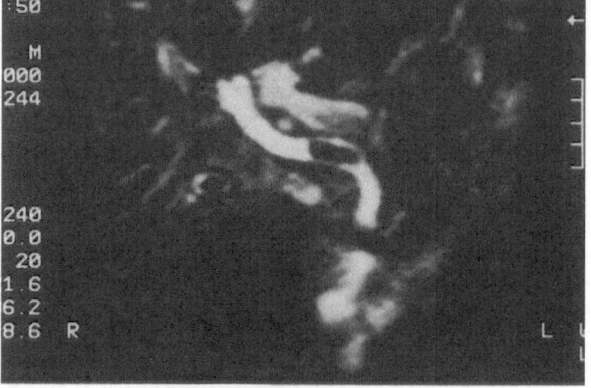

b

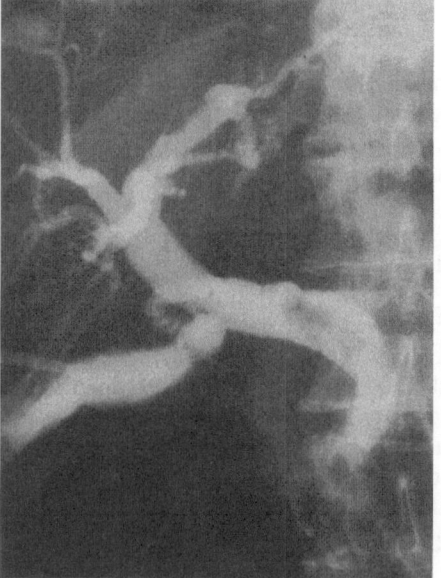

c

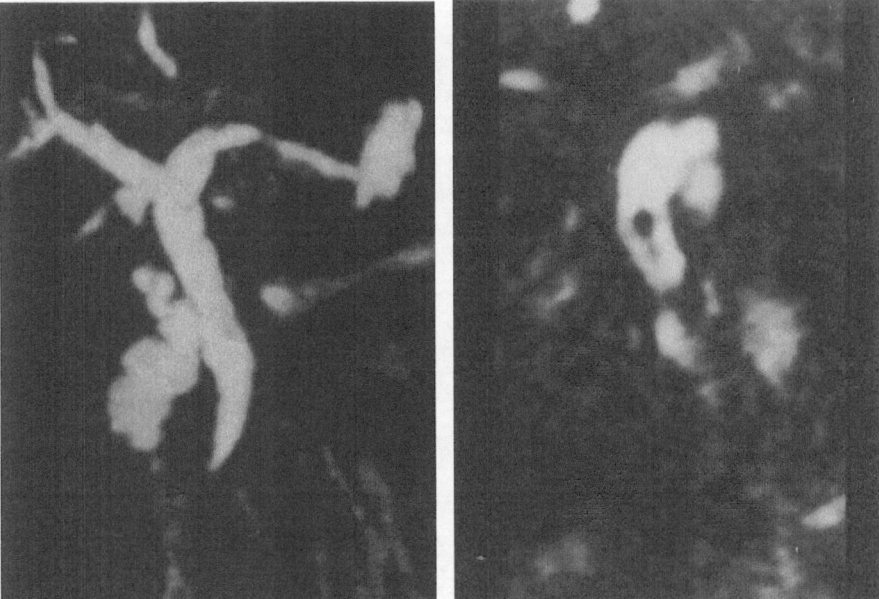

a                                                                                       b

**Fig. 7. a** On MIP-reconstructed image there is no evidence of filling defects. **b** A small stone in the proximal third of the CBD is evident only on source image

### Indications

MRCP should nowadays be considered the diagnostic procedure of choice, if available, for the evaluation of patients with clinical suspicion of CBD after initial screening with ultrasound [17, 18]. In the case of distal stones, MRCP can detect the level of the biliary obstruction and characterize the lesion, allowing a differential diagnosis with other causes of jaundice, as better defined in the chapter on jaundice.

The lack of invasiveness, the absence of contrast media injection, and the three-dimensional images provided, make MRCP particularly valuable, although the higher costs of the procedure, and the limited diffusion of modern equipment with high gradient strength limits the use of MRCP to clinically selected patients. A primary indication is the evaluation of the bile ducts in patients with symptoms compatible with bile duct stones, but with lack of evidence of stones at ultrasound. MRCP is a tool to completely avoid diagnostic ERCP and limit this procedure only to those cases with known biliary stones in order to perform interventional procedures.

### Gallbladder Stones

Ultrasound remains the procedure of choice in the diagnosis of gallbladder stones, with widely known advantages being the low costs and the high sen-

**Fig. 8. a** On MIP image a slight alteration of the signal intensity of the CBD is appreciated. **b** The stone is well evident only on source image

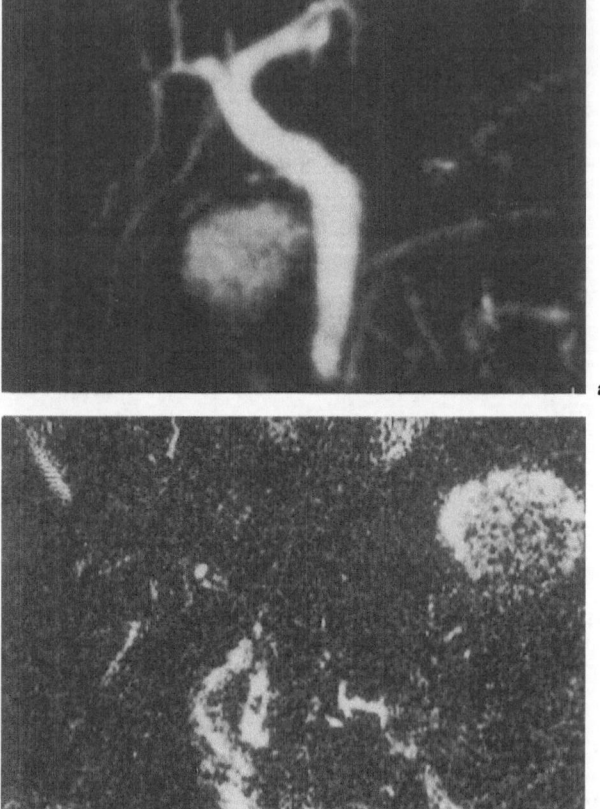

a

b

sitivity and specificity. Although MRCP has no indication for the evaluation of gallbladder stones, it is useful to consider that it may allow the detection of gallbladder stones with the same diagnostic criteria of contrast studies (Fig. 12, 13). Both MIP-recostructed images and single slices must be evaluated for the detection of gallbladder stones. More than in the case of bile ducts stones, small stones can be hidden by the hyperintense content of the lumen in MIP-reconstructed images, but they can be easily detected in single slices.

Besides showing gallbladder stones, with MRCP it is possible to evaluate also the conditions of the wall of the gallbladder, better evident in the axial turbo spin echo T2-weighted images always acquired in conjunction with the MRCP images. In one patient the vanished gallbladder outer margins led us to the diagnosis of an acute cholecystitis, consistent with the symptoms presented by the patient.

Despite the lack of primary indication to the evaluation of gallbladder stones, MRCP may be considered for the evaluation of this group of patients

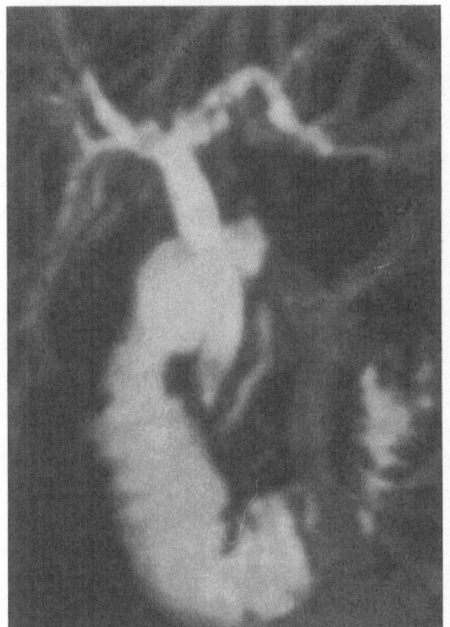

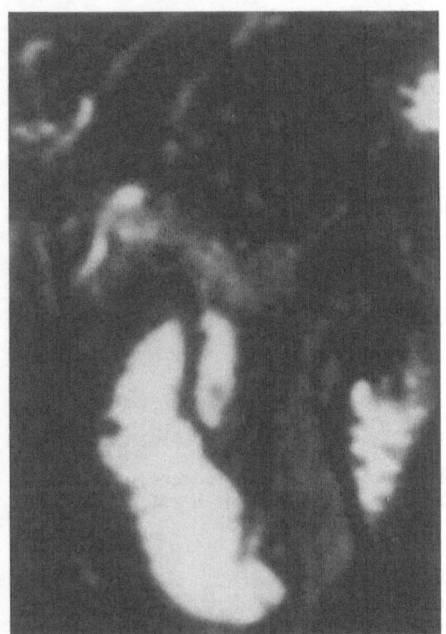

a

b

**Fig. 9a–c.** A 5-mm stone is
not evident on MIP-recon-
structed image (a), but only
on source image (b). c On
ERCP the stone is not
detected on conventional
film due to excessive
filling defect, but it is
extracted with a balloon
catheter

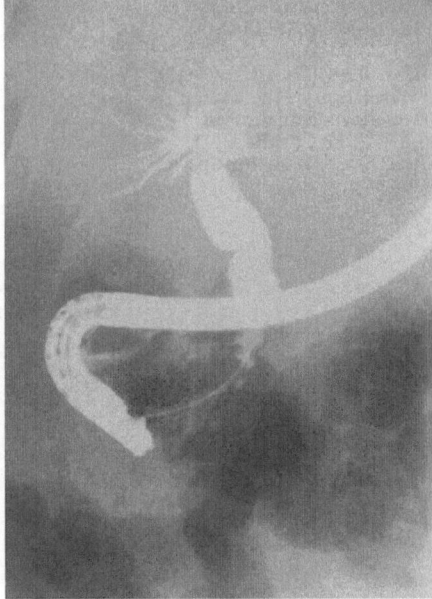

c

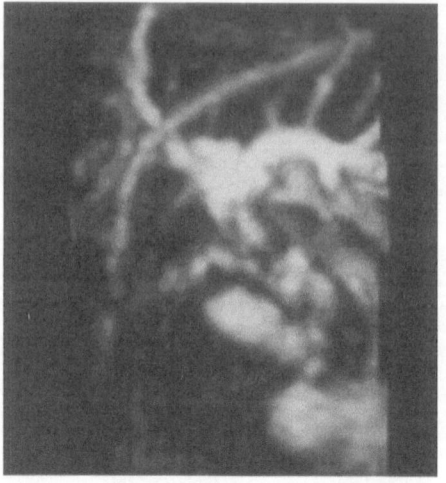
a

**Fig. 10. a** Diffuse inhomogeneous signal in the CBD due to multiple intraluminal stones. **b** Confirmation on ERCP

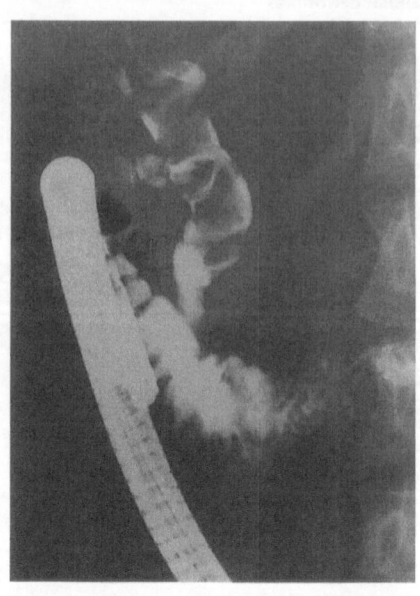
b

**Fig. 11. a, b** On CT scans aerobilia is clearly evident both at the level of the intra-hepatic ducts and at that of the CBD. **c** The air in the CBD causes the inhomogeneous signal in the distal tract of the CBD. **d** However, the evaluation of the source image allows depiction of the distal tract of the CBD, although with poor quality image

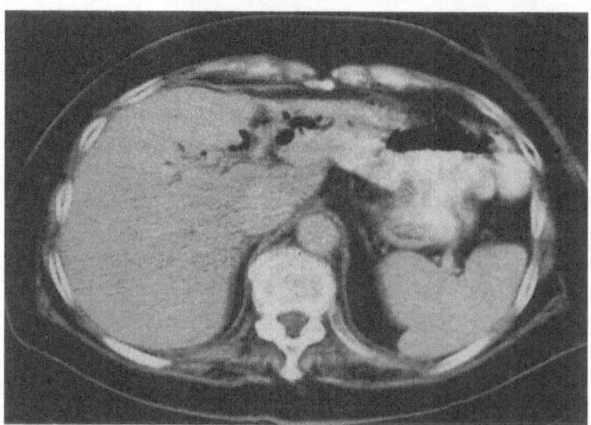
a

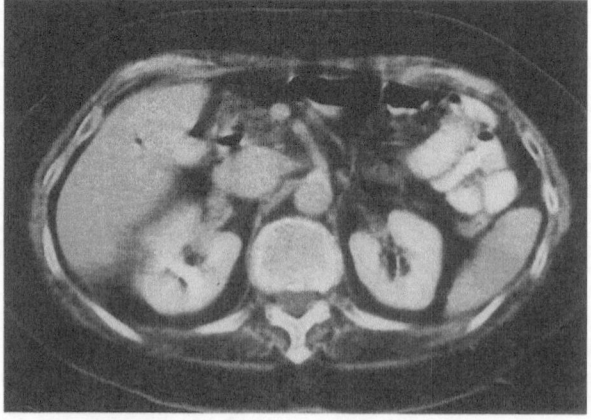
b

**Fig. 11.** (cont.)

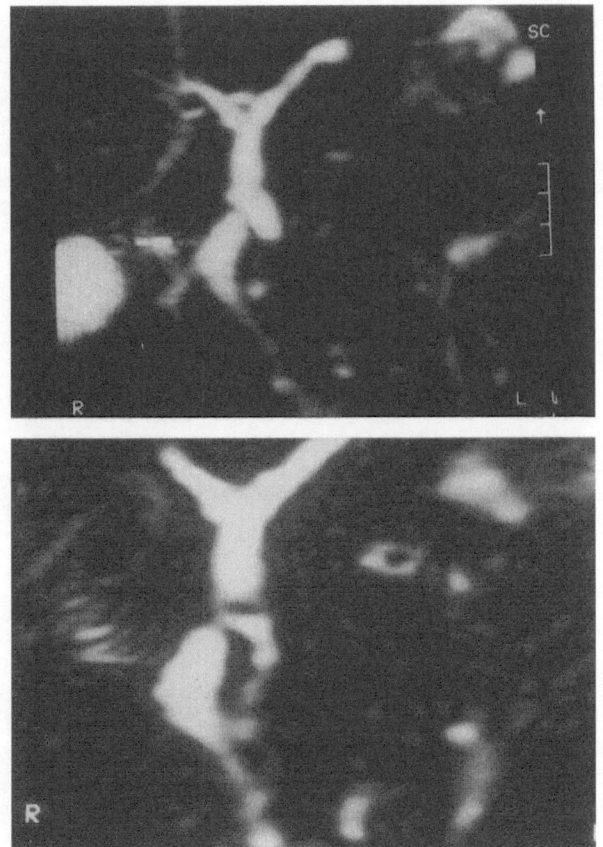

**Fig. 12. a** The gallbladder presents a low signal intensity at the level of the fundus. **b** Multiple stones are well visualized on source image

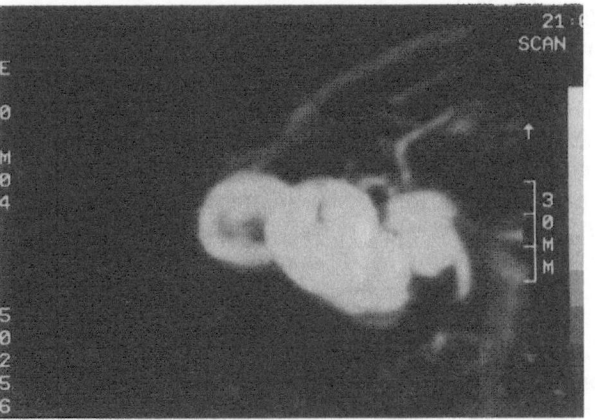

**Fig. 12.** (cont.)

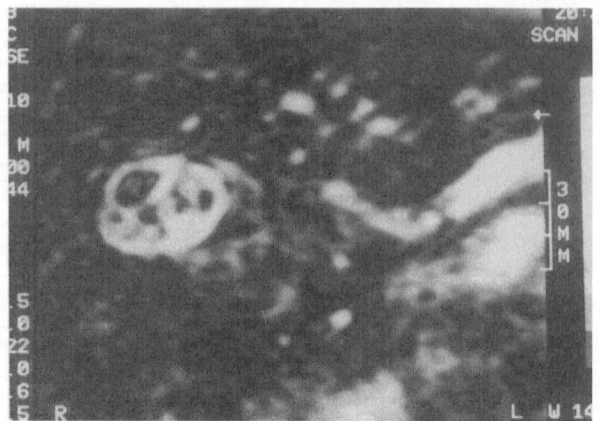

b

**Fig. 13.** Multiple stones in the gallbladder evident even on a MIP-reconstructed image

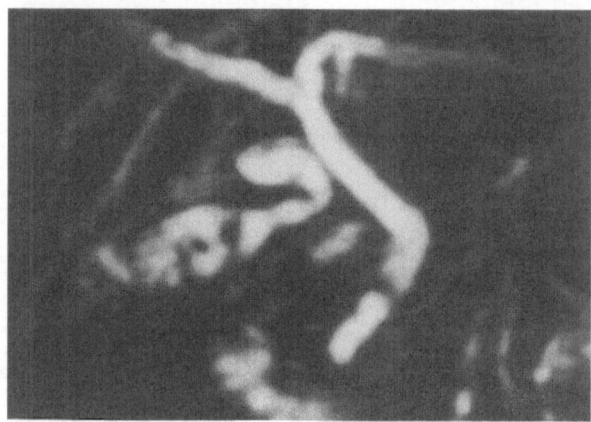

in the preoperative period. MRCP may infact detect associated stones in the CBD, helping to select patients to undergo a therapeutic procedure, either during the laparoscopic cholecystectomy or in a second phase with interventional ERCP [19–21]. A second potential application in the preoperative phase is for the detection of cystic ducts anomalies. Recent work has shown that MRCP may be able to evaluate anomalies of the cystic duct with high accuracy, helping in the guidance of the surgical procedure [22]. Having a complete definition of the anatomy of the patients would limit the potential iatrogenic damage to the CBD, usually occurring in the presence of a short or highly draining cystic duct.

A cost–benefit analysis must be perfomed to define the potential application of MRCP in patients to undergo gallbladder surgery for stone disease. The prevalence of this disease could make the procedure not cost-effective, considering the large number of patients who need to be studied and the increased costs to cure the disease.

# References

1. Reis R, Deutsch AA, Nudelman I, Kott I (1984) Statistical value of various clinical parameters in predicting the presence of choledochal stones. Surg Gynecol Obstet 159:273–276
2. Hauer-Jensen M, Karesen R, Nygaard K, Solheim K, Amlie E et al (1985) Predictive ability of choledocholithiasis indicators: a prospective evaluation. Ann Surg 202:64–68
3. Patel JC, McInnes GC, Bagley JS, Needham G, Krukowski ZH (1993) The role of intravenous cholangiography in pre-operative assessment for laparoscopic cholecystectomy. Br J Radiol 66:1125–1127
4. Shehadi WH, Toniolo G (1980) Adverse reaction to contrast media. Diagn Radiol 137:299–302
5. Pasanen P, Partanen K, Pikkarainen P, Alhava E, Pirinen A, Janatuinen E (1992) ultrasonography, CT and ERCP in the diagnosis of choledocal stones. Acta Radiol 33:53–56
6. Baron RL, Stanley RJ, Lee JKT (1982) Prospective comparison of the evaluation of biliary obstruction using computed tomography and ultrasonography. Radiology 145:91
7. Baron RL (1987) Common bile ducts stones. Reassessment of criteria for CT diagnosis. Radiology 162:419
8. Jeffrey RB, Federle MP, Laing FC, Wall S, Rego J, Moss AA (1983) Computed tomography in choledocolithiasis. AJR 140:1179
9. Franceschi D, Brandt C, Margolin D, Szopa B, Ponsky J, Priebe P, Stellato T, Eckhauser ML (1993) The management of common bile duct stones in patients undergoing laparoscopic cholecystectomy. Am Surg 59:525–532
10. Cotton PB, Lehman G, Vennes J, Geenen JE, Russell RCG et al (1991) Endoscopic sphincterotomy complications and their management: an attempt at consensus. Gastrointest Endosc 37:383–393
11. Grogono JL, Woods WGA (1986) Selective use of operative cholangiography. World J Surg 10:1009–1013
12. Guibaud L, Bret PM, Reinhold C et al (1994) Diagnosis of choledocolithiasis: value of MR cholangiography. AJR 163:847–850
13. Morimoto K, Shimoi M, Shirakawa T et al (1992) Biliary obstruction: evaluation with three-dimensional MR cholangiography. Radiology 183:578–580
14. Guibaud L, Bret PM, Reinhold C et al (1994) Diagnostic accuracy of MR cholangiography in the detection of choledocolithiasis. Radiology 193 (P):134
15. Reinhold C, Bret PM, Guibaud L et al (1994) MR cholangiopancreatography: comparison with Endoscopic Retrograde Cholangiopancreatography. Radiology 193 (P):434
16. Soto JA, Yucel EK, Barish M et al (1994) MR cholangiopancreatography: correlation with endoscopic retrograde cholangiopancreatography. Radiology 193 (P):133
17. Soto JA, Yucel EK, Barish M et al (1994) MR cholangiopancreatography: sequence optimization, new techniques and early clinical experience. Radiology 193 (P):433
18. Hall-Craggs MA, Allen CM, Owens CM et al (1993) MR cholangiography: clinical evaluation in 40 cases. Radiology 189:423–427
19. Mouret P (1991) From the first laparoscopic cholecystectomy to the frontiers of laparoscopic surgery: the future prospectives. Dig Surg 8:124–125
20. Zucker KA, Bailey RW, Gadacz TR, Imbembo AL (1991) Laparoscopic guided cholecystectomy. Am J Surg 161:36–44
21. Schirmer BD, Edge SB, Dix J, Hyser MJ, Hanks JB, Jones RS (1991) Laparoscopic cholecystectomy: treatment of choice for symptomatic cholelithiasis. Ann Surg 6:665–677
22. Taourel P, Bred PM, Reinhold C et al (1995) MR cholangiography. Anatomic variants of the biliary tree. Radiology 197:312

# CHAPTER 6

# MR Cholangiography in Benign Biliary Stenoses

## Introduction

Benign stenoses of the main biliary tract include inflammatory processes of Vater's papilla (papillitis) and iatrogenic stenoses. MR cholangiography can play an important role in the diagnostic evaluation of these patients by allowing a noninvasive study of the main biliary tract.

## Papillitis

Symptoms that arise from diseases of the Oddi's sphincter are similar irrespective of the cause and origin of the obstruction. This condition can result from fibrosis of the papilla or from functional disturbances. However, in both cases the clinical manifestations depend on the sphincteric segment involved [1].

From a clinical standpoint it may be difficult to distinguish papillary stenoses from choledocholitiasis since both conditions can be associated with recurrent pain, either in the right superior quadrant of the abdomen or epigastric. Moreover, both can be associated with laboratory evidence of cholestasis and/or pancreatitis and with dilated main biliary tract or pancreatic duct evident at radiological studies [1, 2].

The primary stenoses result from malformations of the papilla. In addition, chronic and acute inflammatory processes can be responsible for stenoses as well as the adenomiomatosis of the Vater's papilla (similar to the one of the prostatic hypertrophy) [1, 3]. Secondary papillary stenoses can be found in association with cholelitiasis in 26% of cases and with choledocholitiasis in 64%. The mechanism may be either direct, traumatic due to the passage of stones through the sphincter, or due to the continuous irritation of the distal tract of the biliary tree that induces a spasm of the papilla. Together these mechanisms are responsible for 90% of stenoses; another, less frequent cause are previous surgical procedures involving the biliary tree [1].

The common sphincter is the most frequently involved site. Differential diagnosis with the choledocholitiasis is therefore difficult although an isolated stenosis of the biliary sphincter is still possible; a stenosis involving exclusively the pancreatic sphincter is extremely rare [4]. As far as diagnosis is concerned, the stenosis of the papilla can appear on ultrasound as a dilated CBD or pancreatic duct. [5]. Hepatobiliary scintigraphy is a reliable and relatively noninvasive technique for diagnosis of a stenosis of the papilla, given its prolonged (more than 45 min) evaluation of the bile transit up to the duodenum [6].

CT is useful only to exclude pancreatoduodenal malignancies, although this does not rule out a neoplastic process when ultrasound evaluation of the biliary tree is not reliable. Before MR cholangiography ERCP was the only reliable technique for the identification of a papillary stenosis. ERCP allows easy identification of tumors of the Vater's papilla or of the duodenum and the simultaneous performance of papillary biopsies to confirm the diagnosis. An endoscopic sphincterotomy may be necessary to obtain tissue samples. In addition, secretions can be sampled for cytology and manometry of the Oddi's sphincter, and a radiological contrast evaluation to visualize the biliary tract can be performed [1].

### Fibrotic Papillary Stenosis

In the fibrotic papillary stenosis cholangiography usually shows a certain degree of dilatation of the biliary tree associated with a long and smooth or flute-beak-like shrinking of the distal tract of the biliary tree (Fig. 1). A prestenotic dilatation of the ampulla may be present. A delayed drainage of the contrast media at ERCP can support the diagnosis considering that the normal complete drainage time after cholecystectomy is 45 min with the patient in supine position. Opacification of the Wirsung can demonstrate its slight dilatation or no dilatation at all [1, 3].

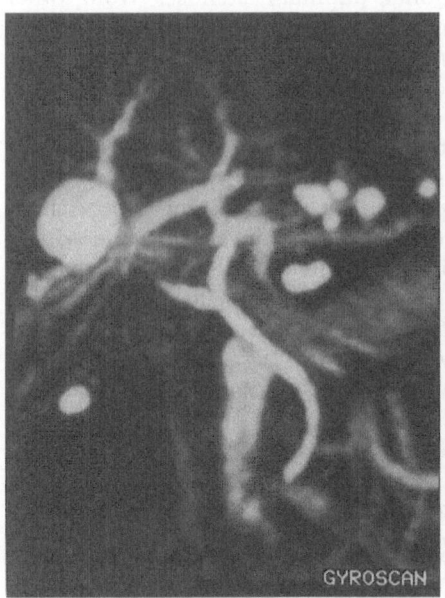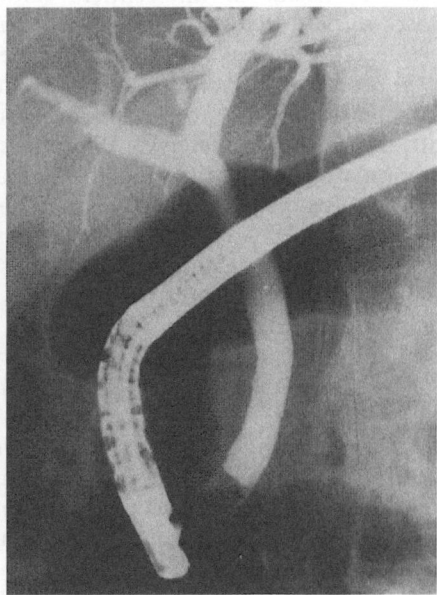

a    b

**Fig. 1. a** MRCP of papillitis with moderately dilated biliary tract that shrinks distally to the flute beak. **b** Similar findings are observed on ERCP

The differential diagnosis between benign and malignant stenoses can be difficult, although complete obstruction usually indicates a malignant stenosis. Glucagon can be necessary for the relaxation of the Oddi's sphincter and for its incannulation as well as to differentiate a spasm from an anatomic stenosis. ERCP is successful in only 82% of cases; for this reason a transhepatic percutaneous cholangiography is sometimes necessary [7]. MR cholangiography allows easy identification of the typical appearance of the biliary tree in fibrotic papillary stenosis. The appearance is that of a dilated biliary tract that shrinks distally to the flute beak (Figs. 2–4). Conventional MR images acquired in the upper abdomen can be important to exclude malignancies of the pancreas and of the main biliary tract.

Drugs that can induce relaxation of the Oddi's sphincter are in progress to differentiate the phlogistic stenosis from the functional spasm. These agents include glucagon and ceruletide, a polipeptide that stimulates the contractile activity of the gallbladder inducing relaxation of Oddi's sphincter. Following the administration of these drugs there is no detention of the biliary tract in cases of phlogistic stenosis of Vater's papilla.

## Functional Papillary Stenoses

Endoscopic manometry of Oddi's sphincter during ERCP can detect phasic contractions of the sphincter that in most cases appear strong, retrograde, and with a paradoxical response to the octapeptide cholecystokinin. Manometry is useful to differentiate functional papillary stenoses from other causes of pain following cholecystectomy [8]. Only a small difference in pressure has been found in functional stenoses compared to phlogistic-fibrotic ones. Moreover, functional stenoses show a nonlinear pressure-endoluminal diameter ratio when the papilla is incannulated and dilated with catheters with increasing diameter [9]. Fibrotic stenoses cannot be evaluated or can be incannulated only with major difficulties.

Recent studies demonstrate that hepatobiliary scintigraphy with technetium ($^{99m}$Tc-IDA) can play a minor role in the noninvasive evaluation of functional and organic papillary stenosis. The signs that define abnormal hepatobiliary scintigraphic findings and support the diagnosis of a papillary stenosis include delayed biliointestinal transit (longer than 1 h), which is the most importat sign, 2-h ductal activity equal to or higher than that of the first hour, the absence of intestinal activity, and an apparent ductal dilatation [10, 11].

At MR cholangiography the appearance of the biliary tract is similar in functional spasms and in fibrotic stenoses. Generally, the dilatation of the biliary is less evident, and pharmacological tests show complete detention of the biliary tract. Endoscopic sphicterotomy is the treatment of papillary stenoses that can be performed in those of fibrotic origin as well as in the functional ones. Following sphicterotomy the outcome is generally satisfactory. A complete resolution of symptoms can be achieved in more than 90% of patients [12]. Accurate follow-up is important considering that restenosis is

**Fig. 2. a** MRCP MIP-reconstructed image shows a wide
dilation of the CBD with a
distal smooth narrowing at
ampulla. **b** A better evaluation is possible on source
image. **c** The axial T2-
weighted image shows only
a hypointense fibrotic tissue
at the level of the papilla

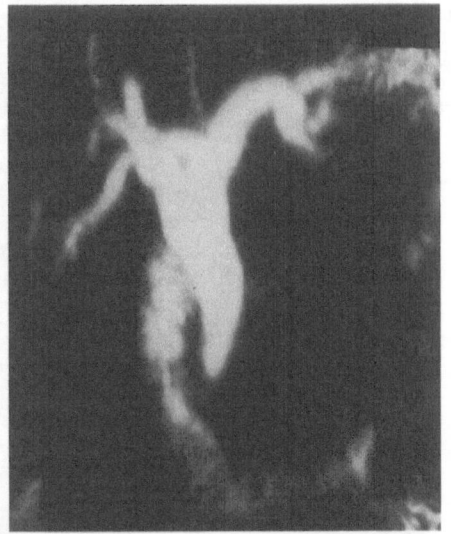

a

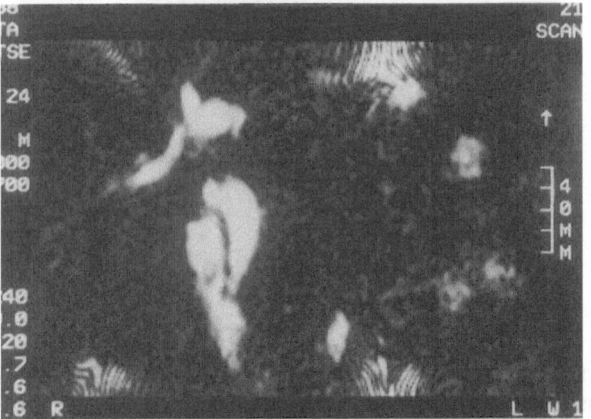

b

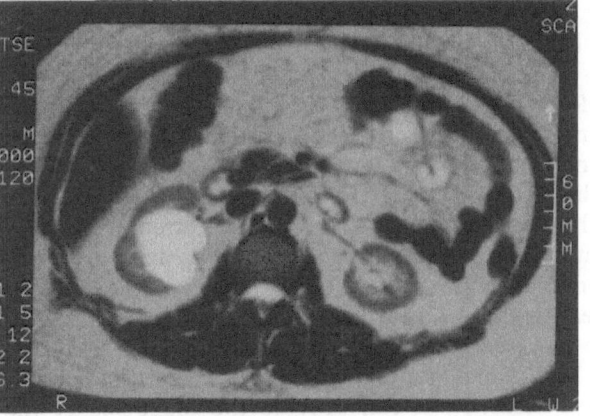

c

**Fig. 3a, b.** Smooth narrowing of the distal tract of the CBD well evaluated both on MIP-reconstructed (a) and source image (b)

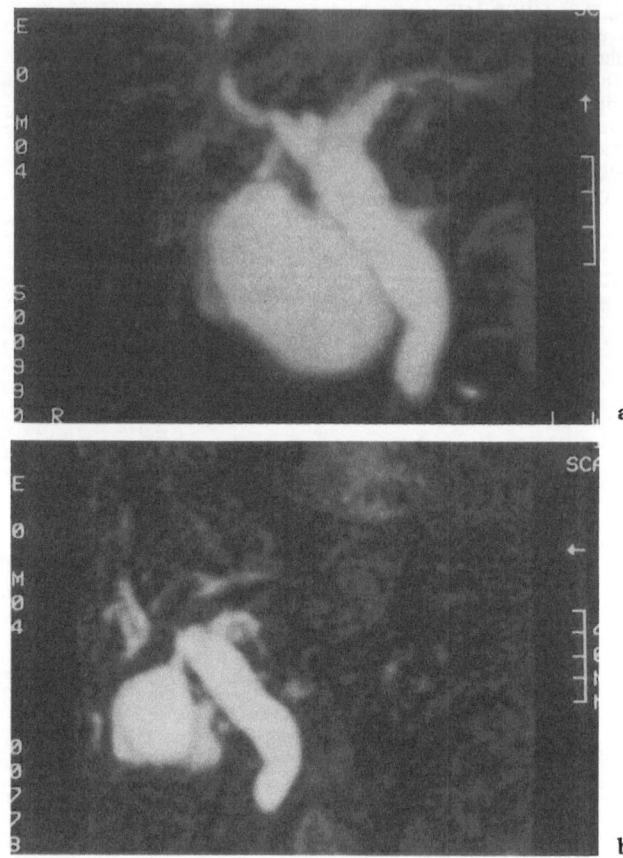

a

b

more frequent after endoscopic sphincterotomy for the fibrotic papillary stenoses (11.5%) than for choledocholitiasis (2.9%) [13].

### Role of MRCP in Phlogistic and Functional Alterations of the Papilla

MRCP may play a very important role in the definition of phlogistic and functional alterations of the papilla. In fact, these clinical entities do not present specific symptoms, and a differential diagnosis must be made with other pathologies of the bile ducts, including stones and neoplasms. A typical presentation is that of a patient, often previously undergoing cholecystectomy, having mild symptoms characterized by recurrent pain or colic or episodes of jaundice. The decision to be made in these patients is whether to treat them (if a morphological alteration is present) or not to treat them (if no morphological alteration is present).

MRCP may provide the correct answer in this group of patients with a high accuracy. It can provide the diagnosis of the presence or absence of

**Fig. 4. a** CT shows a "protruding" tissue at the level of the papilla, compatible with either neoplasm or benign stenosis. **b** MRCP MIP-reconstructed image shows a wide dilation of the CBD with a distal irregular narrowing at ampulla. On ERCP exuberant fibrosis of the papilla was diagnosed

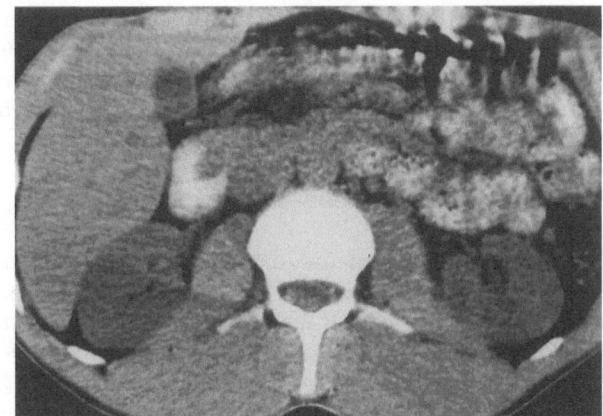

a

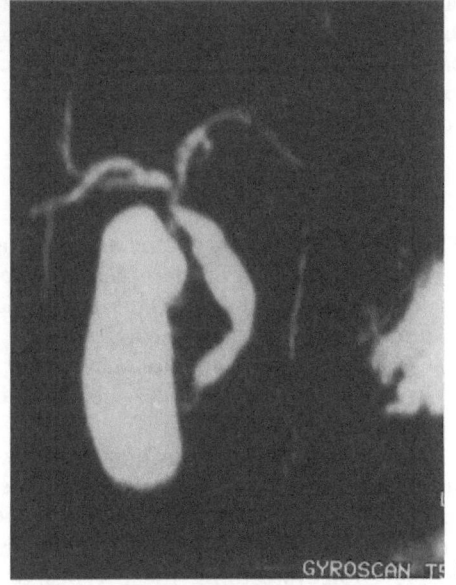

b

stones at first, with an accuracy greater than 90% (see Chap. 5). If the stone is present (fewer than 20% of cases in our experience), ERCP with interventional approach must be performed. If no stones are present, and this is the majority of cases, MRCP provides an accurate evaluation of the biliary anatomy and is able to define the presence of biliary dilatation and the stenosis at papilla. In this group of patients the decision to perform an interventional procedure must be taken according to the degree of the symptoms and to the morphological evidence of the biliary tree on MRCP. Cases with mild symptoms and with no significant dilatation of the bile ducts on MRCP are to be followed up with no intervention. On the other hand, cases with multiple symptoms require manometric evaluation and possibly sphincterotomy.

Including MRCP in the diagnostic protocols therefore limits the role of ERCP to interventional procedures. In our series 20% of cases present stones, and 15%–20% present no stones but symptoms that require treatment by sphincterotomy. More than 60% of cases evaluated by MRCP require no further diagnostic or interventional procedure.

## Iatrogenic Biliary Stenoses

The majority of iatrogenic damages to the extrahepatic biliary tract take place during cholecystectomy. About 20% follow urgent cholecystecomy, with a small percentage from other surgical procedures such as gastric resections [14–16]. More than 90% of benign biliary stenoses are surgically induced. Laparoscopic cholecystectomy, although with short hospitalization time and good esthetic results, shows a slightly higher incidence of complications than laparotomic cholecystectomy. Deziel [22] reported an incidence of stenosis of 0.2%–0.3% following conventional cholecystectomy versus an incidence of 0.6% following laparoscopic cholecystectomy. It is a general opinion that the experience of the operator reduces the risk of complications following laparoscopic cholecystectomy.

### Causes of Bile Duct Injuries

The most common mechanisms of iatrogenic damage are:
- Blind hemostasis or clamping to stop bleeding of the cystic artery, hepatic artery, or portal vein. This either damages directly the hepatic common duct or damages its vascular supply.
- Clamping of the choledochus instead of the cystic duct.
- Excessive traction of the neck of the gallbladder, tenting of the choledochus.

The iatrogenic stenosis may have various causes: lesion of the CBD with surgical repair; cystic duct ligation close to the CBD, with accompanying fibrotic involvement and stenosis of the CBD; excessive retraction of the CBD or hemostasis, with ischemia of the wall of the bile duct. During laparoscopic cholecystectomy these types of problems may be more evident because of misidentification of the CBD as cystic duct, incorrect placement of clips and sutures with resulting fibrosis involving the CBD, or retraction or dissection of the CBD, hemostasis, or electrocautery dissection [17, 18].

Alterations following cholecystectomy are related not only to strictures of the CBD. They can also include minor bile duct injuries, cystic duct leaks, retained CBD stones, and associated biloma or choleperitoneum. All these alterations need to be correctly defined to perform the indicated treatment [19–21].

Damages to the extrahepatic biliary tree are more common when the cystic duct is opposed both to the common hepatic duct and to the right hepatic duct. The resection of an anomalous biliary duct and slippage of the cystic duct ligature must be included in the differential diagnosis of an excessive postsurgery drainage. The drainage resolves spontaneously under these circumstances.

## Treatment of Bile Duct Injuries

The most frequent reparative surgical procedures are various types of bilioenteric anastomoses (choledocho-jejunostomy or hepatico-jejunostomy) since termino-terminal anastomoses present a high incidence of recurrences. Recurrences of biliary stenoses or shrinking of the anastomoses can appear after a symptom-free period of 5–10 years.

If a biliary fistula is present, fistulography with soluble contrast should be the first study to be performed, often demonstrating a biliary stenosis or obstruction. Ultrasound and CT can demonstrate dilated ducts cranially to a stenosis or to a complete ostruction, generally without compression.

In patients with iatrogenic stenosis interventional procedures must be planned either through a percutaneous or an endoscopic approach. Noninvasive imaging of the bile ducts is indicated to define the extent of the lesion and to decide for the most indicated approach for interventional procedure.

**Fig. 5. a** Iatrogenic strictures, following laparoscopic cholecystectomy, located at the proximal third of the CBD within 2-cm from the carrefour (Bismuth type 2). **b** The degree of the stenosis is better evaluated on source image

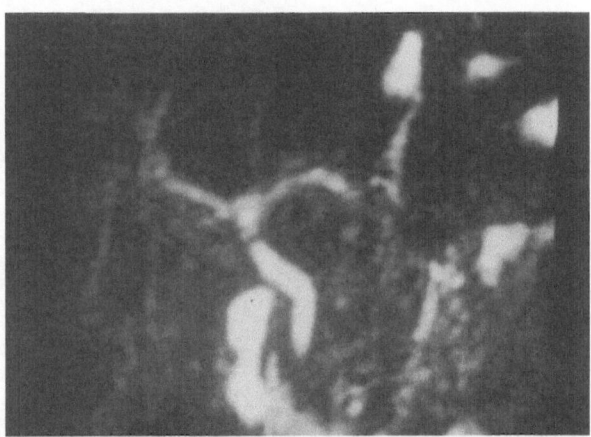

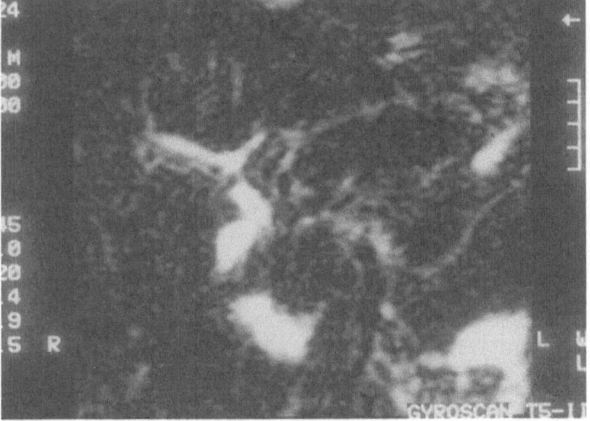

## Diagnostic Evaluation of latrogenic Stenosis: MRCP

Final diagnosis and presurgery mapping are provided by cholangiography performed through the most convenient route. Iatrogenic stenoses are located in the middle portion of the common hepatic duct, are smooth and concentric, and vary in severity from a discrete shrinking to a complete obstruction (Figs. 5–7).

**Fig. 6.** Bismuth type 2 bile duct injury

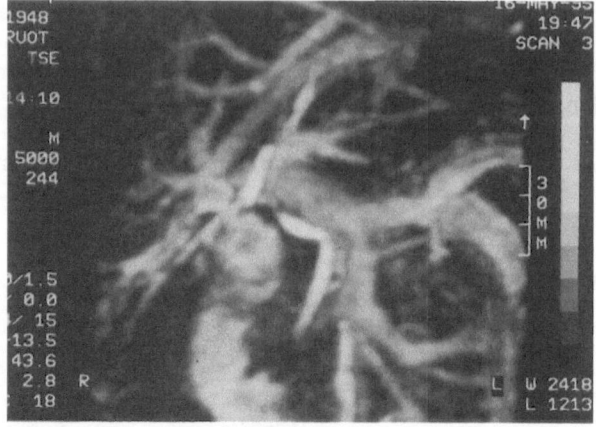

**Fig. 7.** Iatrogenic stricture of the CBD located more than 2 cm from the carrefour (Bismuth type 1)

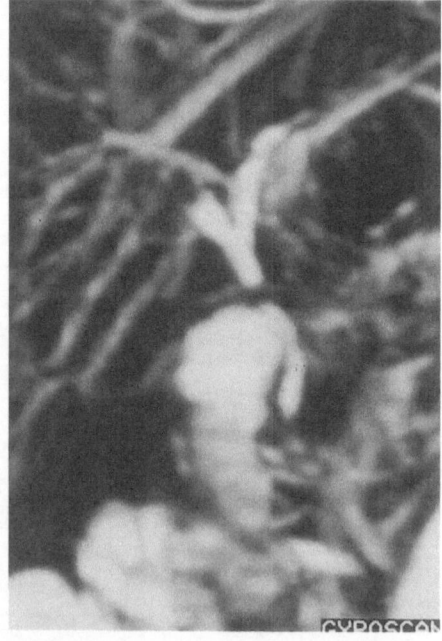

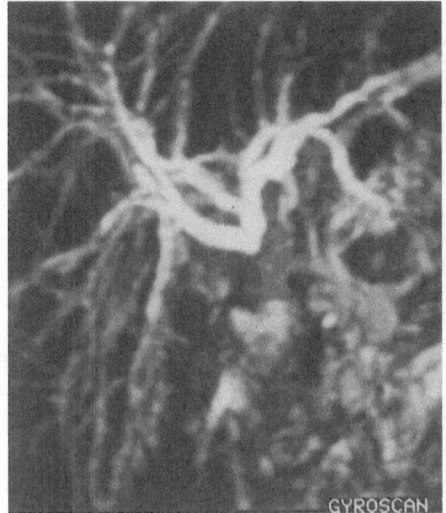
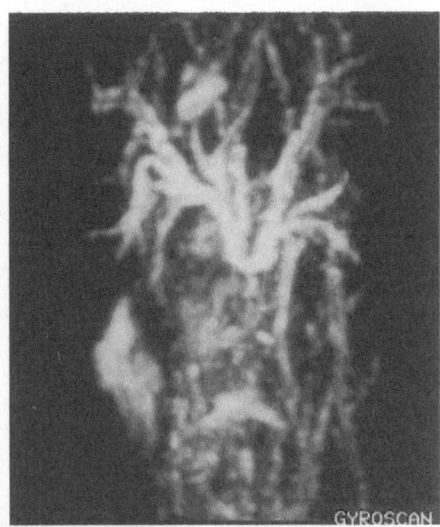

a                                                                                        b

**Fig. 8. a,b** MRCP images on
different rotations correctly
display the dilated intrahepatic ducts and the site
of the obstruction. c The
hepatic stump distal to
the confluence is destroyed,
but the confluence is intact

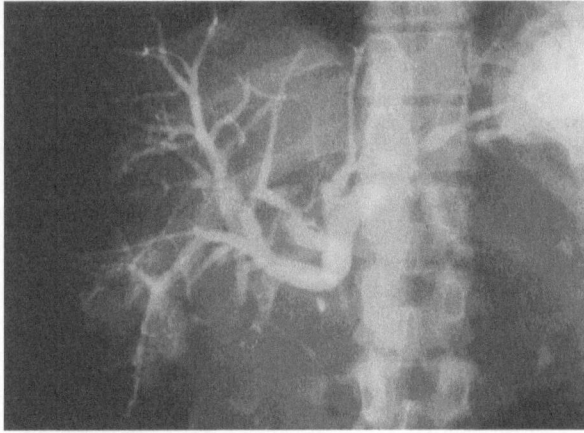

c

Radiologically the stenosis is funnel-shaped or with a distally convex margin while, in case of gallstones, the meniscus sign is present; in some cases
the stenoses can be elongated or irregularly ring-shaped. Clips are often detectable near the stenosis. MR cholangiography provides a complete map of
the bile ducts, showing the dilated segments above the stricture and the presence of the stenosis. Due to the evidence of a very stenotic lumen MRCP
usually overestimates the degree of stenosis, with evidence of obstruction
even in cases with residual patent lumen (Figs. 8, 9).

In conclusion, a stenosis of the middle portion of the common hepatic
duct is usually iatrogenic in patients who undergo surgery for laparoscopic
cholecystectomy. Other rare causes of benign stenosis of the common hepatic duct include inflammations, erosions due to gallstones or other causes.
The evidence of symptoms following laparoscopic cholecystectomy is not al-

**Fig. 9 a–d.** Patient previously have undergone laparoscopic cholecystectomy presented with right upper quadrant pain. On axial T1-weighted (**a**) and T2-weighted (**b**) images an alterated signal intensity is evident, secondary to biliary stasis. **c** MRCP displays both a normal-sized CBD and a dilated accessory duct. **d** Stenosis of the accessory duct is shown also on source image

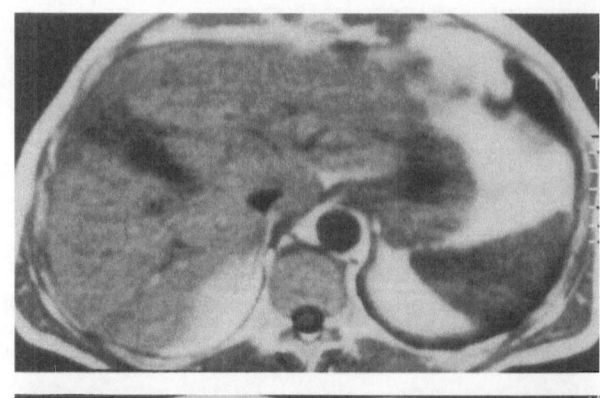

a

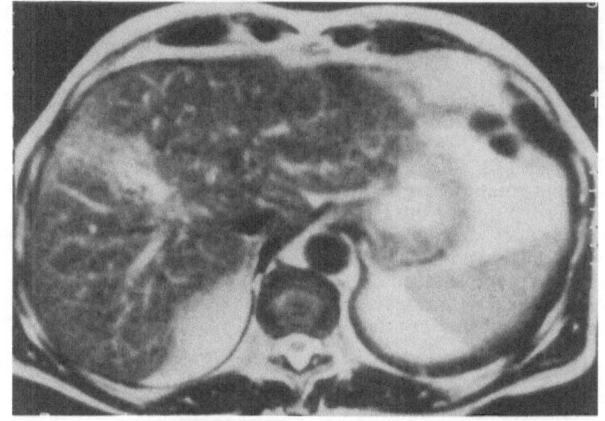

b

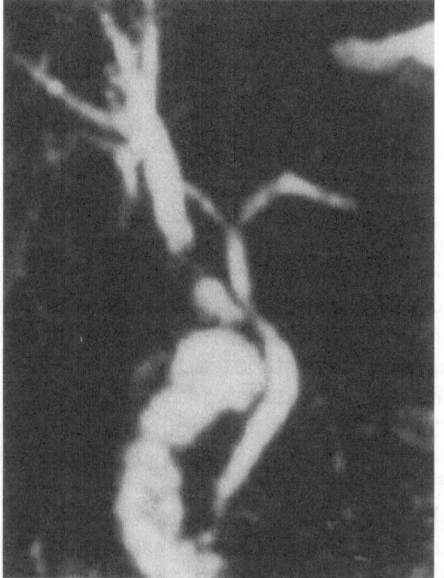

c

**Fig. 9** (cont.)

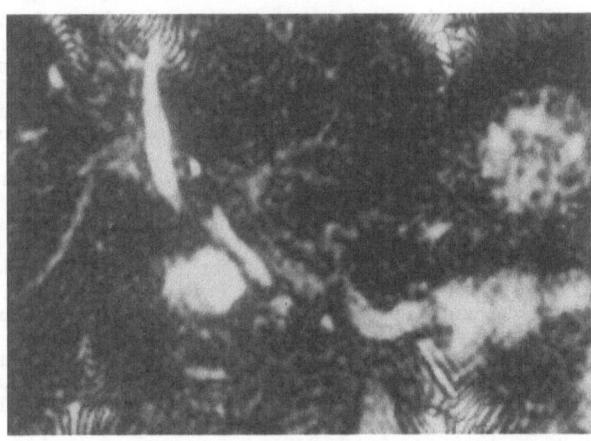

d

ways related to significant stenosis of the common hepatic duct. Other causes may occur, such as residual stones, papillitis, or mild stenotic involvement. In many cases no intervention is required. Therefore MRCP may have an important role in assessing the real clinical entity and in defining the more appropriate therapeutic approach. The complexity of MRCP findings following laparoscopic cholecystectomy is described further in Appendix 2.

## References

1. Classen AM, Leuschner U, Schreiber HW (1983) Stenosis of the papilla Vateri and common duct calculi. Clin Gastroenterol 12:203–214
2. Nardi GL (1973) papillitis and stenosis of the sphincter of Oddi. Surg Clin North Am 53:1149–1160
3. Classen AM (1981) Endoscopic approach to papillary stenosis Endoscopy 13:154–156
4. Albot G (1977) Functional disorders of Oddi's sphincter and of the duodenobiliary systems. In: The sphincter of Oddi: proceedings of the third gastroenterological symposium. Karger, Basel
5. Warhaw AL, Simeone J, Shapiro-RH et al (1985) Objective evaluation of ampullary stenosis with ultrasonography and pancreatic stimulation. Am J Surg 149:65–72
6. Lee RGL, Gregg JA, Koroshetz AM et al (1985) Sphincter of Oddi stenosis: diagnosis using epatobiliary scintigraphy and endoscopic manometry. Radiology 156:793–796
7. Setakis N, Vennart W, Gardner AM, Nayak P (1984) A pre-operative test of the junction of the sphincter of Oddi. Ann R Coll Surg Engl 66:175–178
8. Bortolotti M, calletti GC, Brocchi E et al (1983) Endoscopic manometry of the dioagnosis of the post-cholecystectomy pain sindrome Digestion 28:153–157
9. Hancke E (1981) Intraoperative mural pressure measurements in the papilla of Vater. Langenbecks Arch Chir 354:293–298
10. Lee RGL, Gregg JA, Koroshetz AM et al (1985) Sphincter of Oddi stenosis: diagnosis using epatobiliary scintigraphy and endoscopic manometry. Radiology 156:793–796
11. Zeman RK, Burrel MI, Dobbins J (1985) Post cholecystectomy syndrome: evaliuation using biliary scintigraphy and endoscopic retrograde cholangiopancreatography. Radiology 156:787–792
12. Rosch W, Reimann JF, Lux G, Linder HG (1983) Long-term follow up after endoscopic sphincterotomy. Endoscopy 13:152–153
13. Ell CH, Geocze ST, Riemann JF (1984) Successful endoscopic traetment of extensive recurrent papillary stenosis six years after endoscopic papillotomy. Endoscopy 16:246–248

14. Andren-Sandberg A, Johansson S, Bengmark S (1985) Accidental lesion of the common bile duct at cholecystectomy. II. Results of treatment. Ann Surg 201:452–455
15. Southern Surgeons Club (1991) A prospective analysis of 1518 laparoscopic cholecystectomies. N Engl J Med 324:1073–1078
16. Ghahremany GG, Crampton AR, Bernstein JR, Caprini JA (1991) Iatrogenic biliary tract complications: radiological features and clinical significance. 11:441–456
17. Andren-Sandberg A, Johansson S, Bengmark S (1985) Accidental lesion of the common bile duct at cholecystectomy. II. Results of treatment. Ann Surg 201:452–455
18. Ghahremany GG, Crampton AR, Bernstein JR, Caprini JA (1991) Iatrogenic biliary tract complications: radiological features and clinical significance. 11:441–456
19. Chartrand-lefevre C, Dufresne MP, Lafortune M et al (1994) iatrogenic injury to the bile duct: a working classification for radiologists. Radiology 193:523–526
20. Christensen RA, van Sonnenberg E, Nemcek AA Jr et al (1992) Inadvertent ligation of the aberrant right hepatic duct at cholecystectomy: radiological diagnosis and therapy. Radiology 1993:549–553
21. Trerotola SO, Savander SJ, Lund GB et al (1992) Biliary tract complication following laparoscopic cholacystectomy: imaging and intervention. Radiology 184:195–200
22. Deziel DJ, Millikan KW, Economou SG, Doolas A, Ko ST, Airan MC (1993) Complications of laparoscopic cholecystectomy: a national survey of 4292 hospitals and an analysis of 77604 cases. Am J Surg 165 (1):9–14

# CHAPTER 7

# Involvement of Biliary System by Malignant Neoplasm

## Introduction

Biliary involvement in the course of a malignant neoplasm occurs frequently and constitutes an important clinical event [1]. The involvement can be direct when the neoplasm origins from a biliary duct, such as cholangiocarcinomas or gallbladder carcinoma, or indirect when there is biliary duct compression by nonbiliary neoplastic lesions, such as pancreas carcinomas, subhilar hepatic lymphoadenopathies, and metastatic hepatic lesions compressing segmental biliary ducts [2–4].

This chapter evaluates the MR cholangiography findings detectable in case of malignant neoplasm [5]. As explained in Chap. 4, MR cholangiography cannot be considered as an isolated modality in this field. Regarding lesion definition, characterization, and staging the information from conventional (T1- and T2-weighted) MR images are very important [6]. Therefore morphological findings in these images are also discussed in this chapter. MR diagnostic examination of the biliary system must be considered a single examination, made by both MR cholangiography sequences and conventional ones.

## Carcinoma of the Pancreas

Pancreatic carcinoma is the most frequent cause of obstructive jaundice (26%–47% in various studies). The head of the pancreas, with biliary involvement, is the most common site (70%), whereas the adenocarcinoma is the most frequent histological type (85% of cases). Over the past 40 years its incidence has tripled, although this seems to have reached a plateau since the 1980s. In this disease there are no certain predisposing factors. However, excessive smoke, alcohol, and coffee seems to be predisposing factors [7]. Moreover, there is a tendency to consider chronic pancreatitis as a favoring factor, even in the lack of morphological verification [8, 9].

Besides jaundice, the most frequent symptoms are loss of weight, pain, nausea, and vomiting. Moreover, in addition to the bilirubin increase, there is very often increased alkaline phosphatase, transaminase, and hematic lipase. The pancreatic carcinoma marker is CA 19-9, although its sensitivity and specificity must still be validated to propose its use in screening.

Survival is correlated to the stage at the time of the diagnosis but is very low (1% after 5 years from diagnosis). Stage 1 corresponds to a neoplasm confined to the pancreas, stage 2 presents locoregional lymphoadenopathy, and in stage 3 there is peripancreatic structures infiltration (involvement) or metastasis. Only 5% of patients are in stage 1 at diagnosis [10].

It is necessary to provide a separate description for the ampullar carcinoma, which is associated with a higher survival rate (26%). The difference between an ampullar carcinoma and a pancreatic carcinoma infiltrating the ampulla is obtained by an accurate histological examination. In diagnostic imaging these entities are considered undistinguished, and the single term of periampullar area carcinoma is used to define it. Only in noninfiltrating duodenum and pancreas neoplasm is the term of intrampullar carcinoma used. The lesions interesting ampulla and periampullar area (which are the most frequent events) are called mixed lesions.

## MR Cholangiography of the Pancreatic Carcinoma

### Biliary Ducts

MR cholangiography images demonstrate clearly the biliary involvement from neoplasm [11]. The CBD appears dilatated, with complete occlusion of the middle or distal third, at the level of the intrapancreatic tract. The classical morphological aspect of biliary oclusion by pancratic carcinoma is defined by the "mouse tail" pattern, with short segmental occlusion. This aspect can also be detected by MR cholangiography, despite limitations due to the reduced spatial resolution. In general, a sudden interruption of the biliary dilatation is a sign of carcinoma of the pancreas, although is not very specific (Fig. 1). In MR cholangiocolangiography it is often possible to observe the nipple's mark (sign), a little biliary niche stretching downstream, at the occlusion level (Fig. 2).

In the case of a long lasting dilatation, often in old patients with large tumors, the dilated CBD assumes a tortuous aspect, with a preocclusive horizontal tract. In the presence of a polypoid process projecting in the lumen at the biliary occlusion level the ampullar lesions can be diagnosed. In our experience, we do not find these aspects on MR cholangiography images. However, as in case of CBD stone, an intraluminal lesion can be evaluated in detail with MR cholangiography.

### Pancreatic Duct

The morphological aspect of the pancreatic duct dilatation in ERCP is important in the differential diagnosis between pancreatitis and neoplasm [12, 13]. These aspects, which are used even in semeiotics of the Wirsung's dilatation in CT, are also valuable in MR cholangiography. The occlusion from neoplasm presents a morphology such as the biliary occlusion, with a "mouse tail" pattern, or generally, with sudden reduction in duct size. On the other hand, in pancreatitis a longer stenosis is present, with a homogeneous as-

**Fig. 1a, b.** Pancreatic head carcinoma. **a** MRCP image shows a sudden interruption of the CBD with concomitant dilatation of the Wirsung duct. **b** On T1-weighted axial MR image the hypointense mass is clearly seen

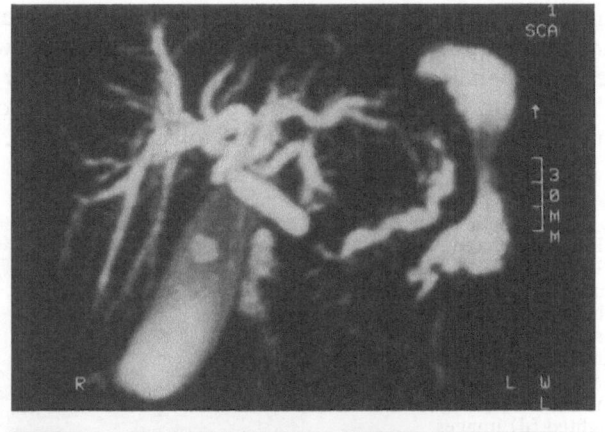

a

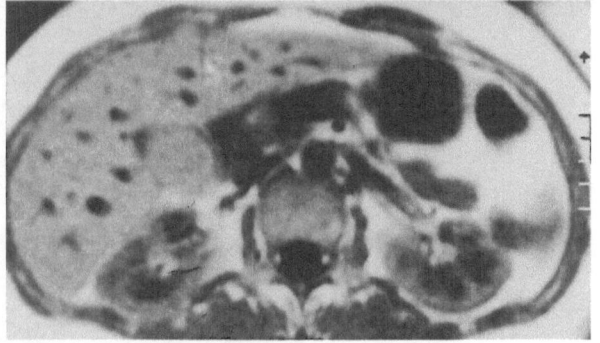

b

pect. The morphological aspects of the ductal dilatation are also important. In neoplasm the duct cranially to the dilatation is homogeneously dilated, whereas in chronic pancreatitis an irregular dilatation, with a beaded pattern, alternating dilated and stenotic segments, is present (Figs. 3, 4).

During ERCP a relative stenosis (encasement), with or without modest duct dilation upstream is sometimes present. It is probable that this aspect is hard to interpret by MR cholangiography due to the reduced spatial resolution, but the possibility to identify the neoplatic lesion on T1 and T2-weighted images provides high sensitivity.

Lesions of the pancreatic head hardly reach large dimensions and never present a central excavation. If this occurs, a cavity communicating with the pancreatic duct can be detected. MR cholangiography findings would be superimposed onto those of a pseudocyst, with very irregular walls.

### MR Conventional Images

As pointed out above, in neoplastic disease MR conventional images must be acquired in association with MR cholangiography in order to identify and stage the lesion. T1-weighted images (with low TR and TE to increase the in-

trinsic contrast), T2-weighted images (with turbo spin echo technique to reduce acquisition time) and fat suppression images, which allow to improve
the focal pancreatic lesions' evaluation, are all very important. With high
field strength equipment, the use of a contrast agent can be helpful, with dynamic evaluations after intravenous injection [14, 15].

**Fig. 2 a–d.** Nipple's sign. a
MIP-reconstructed MRCP
image showing a wide dilation of the CBD and the intrahepatic ducts. b Nipple's
sign is better appreciated on
source image. c–d The pancreatic carcinoma is well evident on T1- (c) and T2-
weighted (d) images

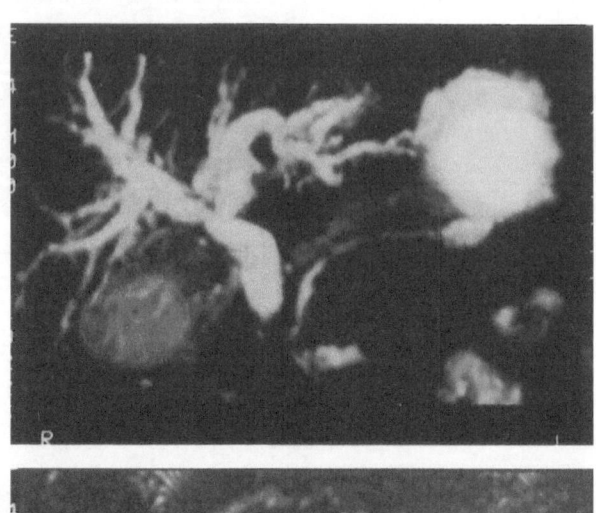

a

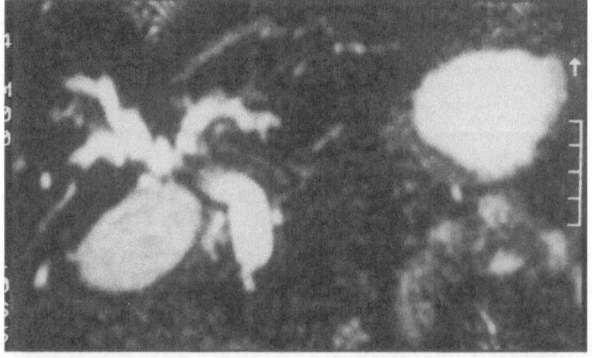

b

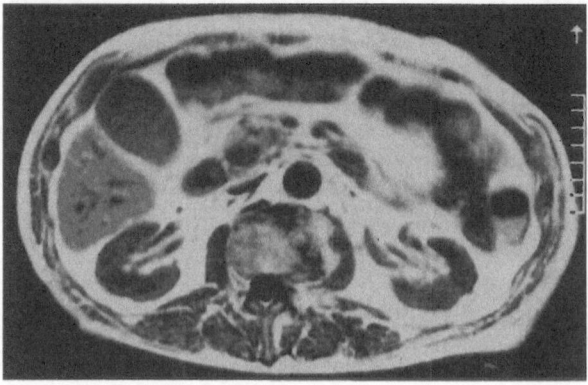

c

**Fig. 2** (cont.)

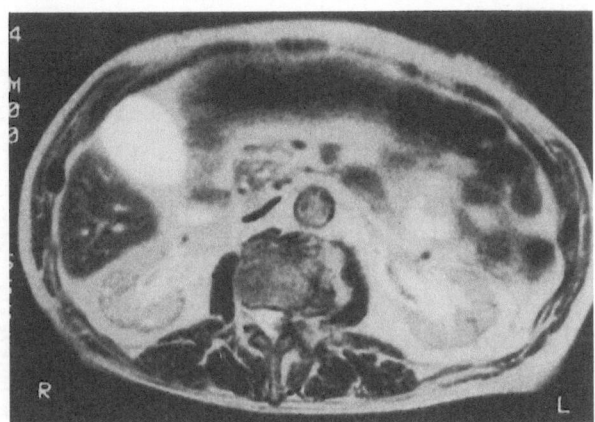

d

## Lesion Identification

Pancreatic carcinoma presents as a clearly low signal intensity lesion on T1-weighted images and slightly high signal intensity on T2-weighted images due to the prolongated T1 and T2 of the surrounding pancreatic parenchyma. Particularly with medium-field equipment on T1-weighted images the lesion is identified with high accuracy and only in the presence of a significant epineoplastic pancreatitis, the delineation of the neoplasm margins may be difficult. In MR the high intrinsic contrast identifies lesions of 2 cm or lower and, theoretically, even smaller lesions such as in the case of pancreatic insulinomas [16]. In theory, also in pancreatic adenocarcinoma we could detect smaller lesions; however, the absence of symptoms does not allow evaluation of patients affected with pancreas adenocarcinoma in more earlier stages.

Also in absence of pancreatic margin irregularities it is possible to demonstrate the lesion clearly as an area of low signal intensity on T1-weighted

**Fig. 3. a** Sudden occlusion of the Wirsung duct with homogeneous dilation of the duct. **b** ERCP image confirming MRCP findings. **c** T1-weighted axial image depicting the hypointense mass at the level of the head of the pancreas

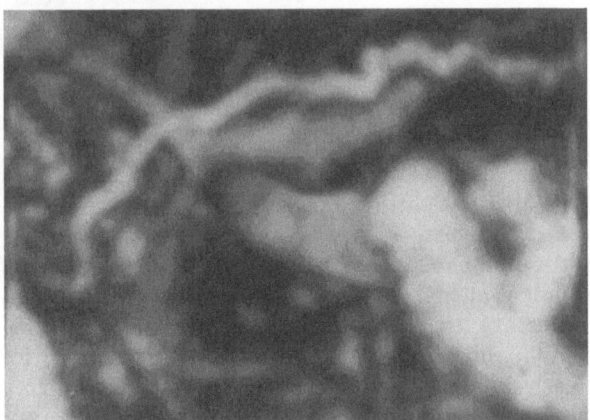

a

**Fig. 3.** (cont.)

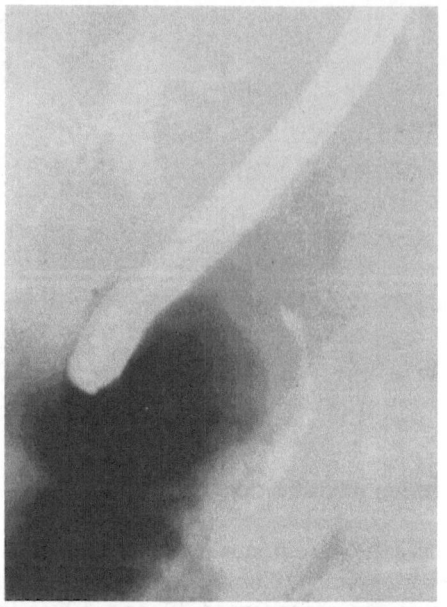

b

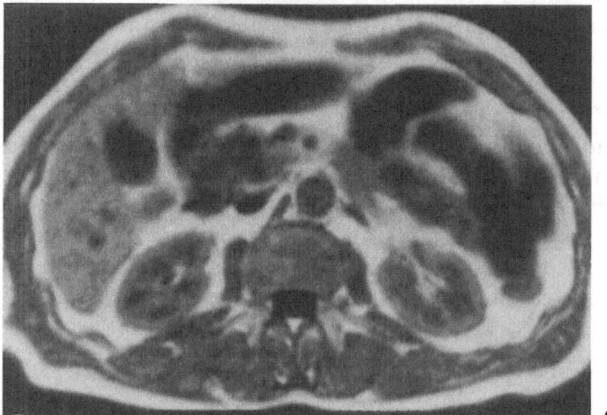

c

images in comparison with surrounding parenchyma (Fig. 5). In our study the smallest identified lesion was located at the level of the uncinate (hooked) process, with a 15-mm diameter. Although T2-weighted images demonstrate the neoplastic lesion, they present an inferior intrinsic contrast. Equipment at high field provides inferior results on T1 images. In this case it is necessary to complete the examination with fat suppression images or with dynamic studies after contrast agents injection which demonstrate in the early phase an area of low signal intensity corresponding to the pancreatic lesion in comparison with the surrounding parenchyma [17].

**Fig. 4a–c.** Pancreatic head carcinoma. **a** MRCP image with homogeneous dilation of the Wirsung duct. **b, c** Axial T1- (**b**) and T2-weighted (**c**) images showing the pancreatic mass

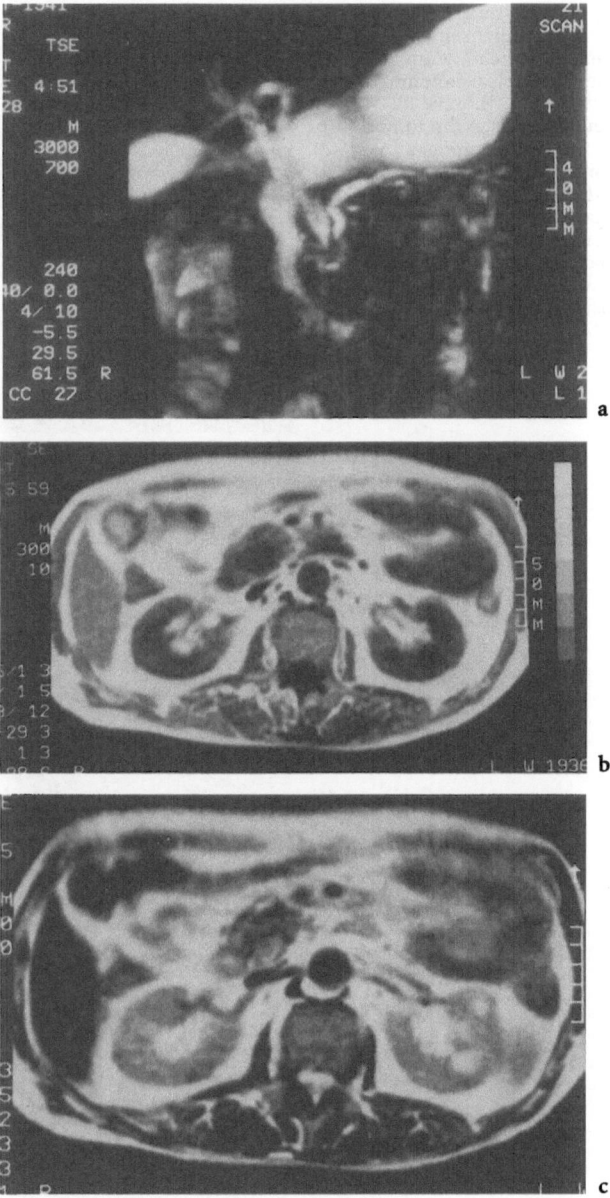

Larger lesions determine a pancreatic margin irregularity, or a volumetric increase in the pancreatic head. It is to remember that in older patients pancreatic atrophy is present and a pancreatic head that presents with apparently regular dimensions it has really an increased volume, in comparison with the atrophic parenchyma.

**Fig. 5. a** CT image showing the enlargement of the pancreatic head, without densitometrical inhomogeneities. **b** On axial T1-weighted image the tumor is clearly evident, as a hypointense lesion closing to the duodenum. **c** MRCP image showing compression of the CBD, rather than infitration. At surgery it was a malignant somatostatinoma

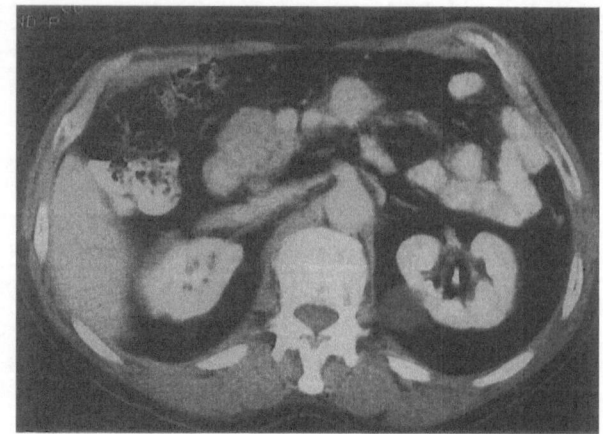

a

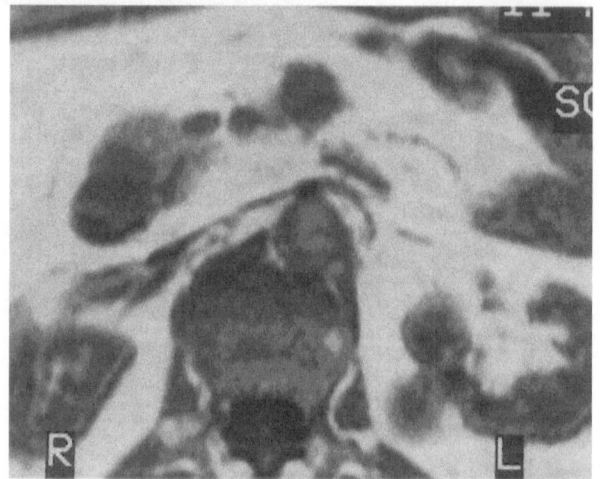

b

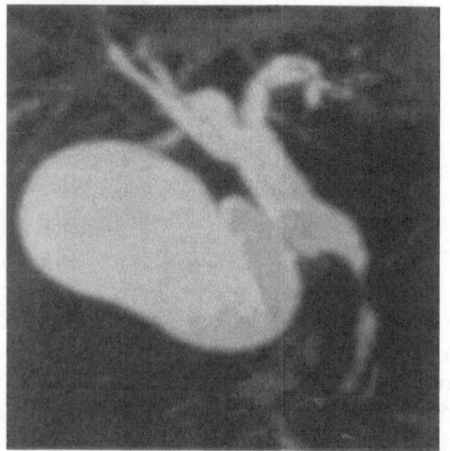

c

While these considerations in CT are very important, in MR they lose their significance. The pancreatic lesion can be differentiated from other pancreatic portions in relation to the signal intensity differences (low signal intensity in the neoplasms, higher in pancreatic atrophy in relation to the adipose cell presence due to fat substitution of normal parenchyma). In lesions involving the uncinate process, the obliteration of the fat tissue surrounding the mesenteric vessels can be evaluated, in addition to the neoplasm definition.

## Staging

In staging pancreatic carcinoma it is necessary to evaluate the retroperitoneal extension towards the peripancreatic fatty tissues, the vascular infiltration, the lymphoadenopathy, and the metastases [18]. Retroperitoneal infiltration can be clearly documented on MR images, although patients with larger lesions often show reduced fatty tissue due to a neoplastic cachectic state. The extension towards the perivascular fatty tissue, particularly perimesenteric and near to the celiac tripode, suggests a pancreatic lesion in advanced stage.

The infiltration of the main peripancreatic vessels is a mark of lesion unresectability. In the presence of simple contact between the lesion and the vessel without size reduction the hypothesis can be considered that there is no vascular infiltration. This finding is not specific since often at the moment of the surgical operation adventitious infiltration is demonstrated. The contact indicates unresectability if it is with the aorta, caval vein, or arterial structures (superior mesenteric artery or celiac tripode). On the other hand, with the absence of a fat plane and the contact of the tumor with the superior mesenteric vein (a frequent finding in the pancreatic head's lesions) the lesion can be considered potentially resectable.

The presence of large expansive processes often causes occlusion of various vessels; their nonvisualization on MR conventional images indicates their involvement from neoplasm. Vessels still patent but completely surrounded from neoplasm and with a reduced size must be considered involved.

As regards the evaluation of vascular involvement, MR angiographic images can be associated with the MR conventional images. We use the phase contrast technique with cardiosynchronization to obtain high-quality images of the arterial and venous structures. On these images it is possible to define vascular occlusion, and also more subtle diagnostic findings, with identification of the vascular encasement of the main peripancreatic branches and gastroduodenal artery.

MR identifies the lymphoadenopathy with the same signal intensity of the primary neoplastic lesion. In 15%–30% of cases increased lymph nodes are individualized. The most frequent site of lymphoadenopathies is at the level of the hilar hepatic region, the porto-caval space, or near the primary mass in the retroperitoneum. Metastases of the pancreas carcinoma develop at the hepatic level.

Various studies have shown that, as regards the identification of repetitive hepatic lesions, MR sensitivity is equal to or slightly higher than that of CT [19]. In the near future these data will probably be improved thanks to the use of hepatic organ-specific contrat agents, in this moment in advanced phase of clinical validation (Gd-BOPTA, Mn-DPDP, Gd-EOB, Gd-DTPA).

## Cholangiocarcinoma

Cholangiocarcinoma is a rare neoplasm. The clinical manifestation is obviously jaundice in view of biliary pertinence of the neoplasm [20]. The early symptoms allow diagnosis of very small lesions, and the slow growth justifies high survival of this neoplasm. Particularly carcinomas situated at the level of the CBD have a good prognosis while those located at the confluence have a poor prognosis due to the earlier development of biliary complications.

The sites of involvement are as follows: CBD (30%–36%), common hepatic duct (15%–30%), hepatic ducts confluence, with the classic pattern of Klatskin's tumor (10%–26%), and intrahepatic ducts (8%–13%). The most frequent pathological pattern is the scirrhous one, often without mass evidence, but with infiltration of the biliary duct. Sometimes differentiation is difficult from a sclerosing cholangitis. Rarely the neoplasm presents as a papillar process projecting into the biliary lumen. In intrahepatic duct neoplasm the nodular type can develop, with an expansive process infiltrating the biliary ducts and extending at the level of the surrounding hepatic parenchyma [1, 21].

### MR Cholangiography

MR cholangiography in cholangiocarcinomas is characterized by the presence of a sudden biliary occlusion, with marked dilatation of the biliary system. Images clearly demonstrate the level of biliary occlusion, with visualization of regular size biliary ducts downstream (Fig. 6). It is possible to evaluate the biliary stenosis extension, calculating the distance between two biliary segments, dilatated upstream and regular downstream, and this provides information about lesion dimension (Fig. 7).

The occlusion is represented mainly by sudden interruption of the biliary ducts due to a infiltrating scirrhous neoplastic disease, the most frequent pattern of biliary neoplasm. In very rare vegetating forms the morphology of the lesion projecting into the lumen can be evaluated with MR cholangiography, as well as in the case of biliary stones [22].

In the CBD stenosis the relationship of the stenosis with the cystic duct is evaluated. Although visualization of the cystic duct is insufficient, the cystic duct level can be identified in relation to the gall bladder dilatation (the dilatated gall bladder corresponds to an involvement at the level of or caudal to the cystic duct).

In Klatskin's tumor it is necessary to assess whether there is a biliary duct interruption at the level of the common hepatic duct, downstream from the

**Fig. 6a–c.** Klatskin tumor.
**a** ERCP image, after placement of a drainage shows a
Klatskin tumor; on this
projection the carrefour is
not visible. **b** MRCP image
with the same view as ERCP
offers a comparable evaluation of the intrahepatic bile
ducts. **c** MRCP allows rotation of the image, providing
a better visualization of the
carrefour

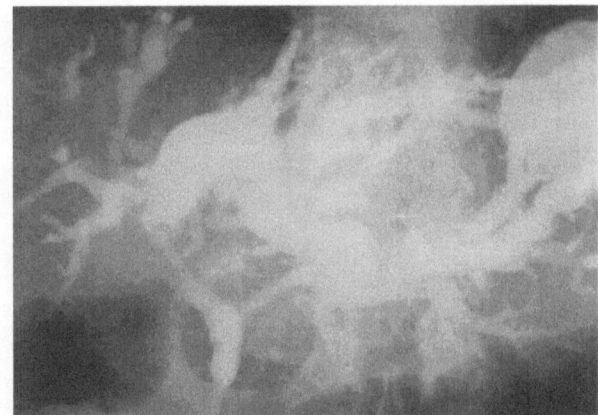

a

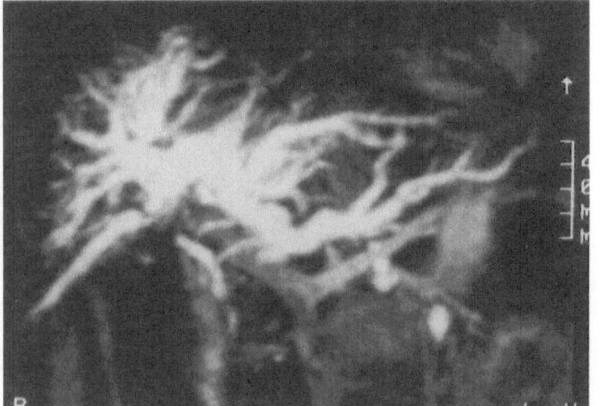

b

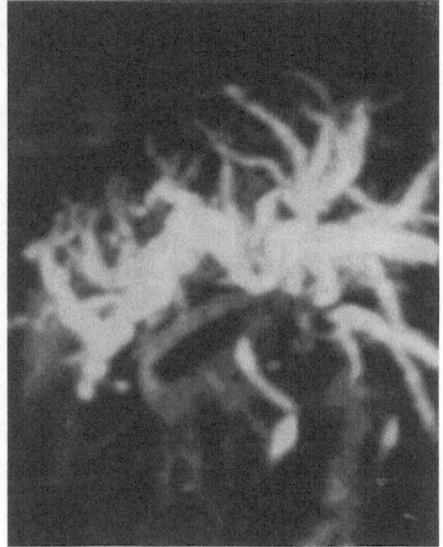

c

**Fig. 7a–c.** Recurrent cholangiocarcinoma in a patient previously treated with bilioenteric anastomosis. a MRCP shows the dilated intrahepatic ducts and the sudden occlusion at the level of the anastomosis. b The source image better depicts the sudden stenosis. c On the axial T1-weighted image the hypointense mass is well evaluated

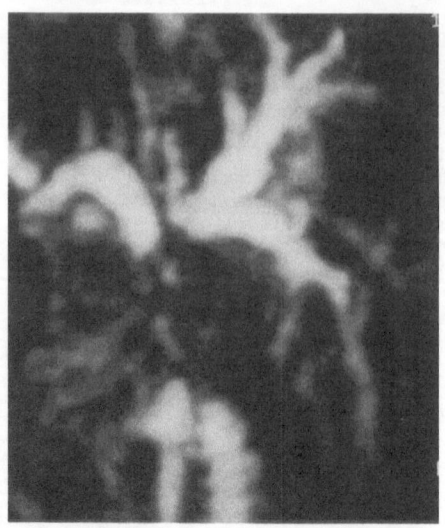

a

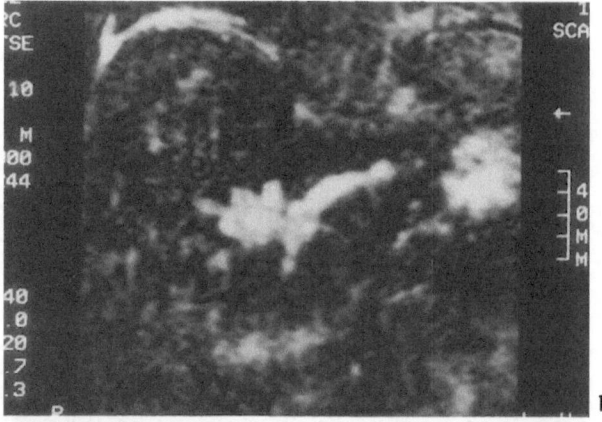

b

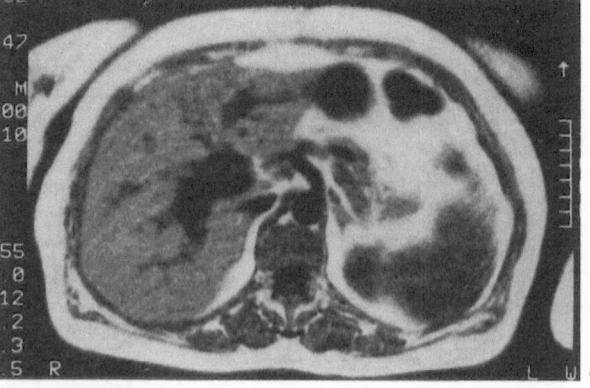

c

confluence, or whether there is involvement upstream, with separation of the right and left ducts or even of the single intrahepatic segmental ducts. The consequences are obvious in the choice of a therapeutic approach.

## MR Conventional Images

T1- and T2-weighted MR images are very important for assessing the neoplastic lesions. The lesion nature does not allow in every case the clear identification of an expansive process. In infiltrating scirrhous lesions it is generally not possible to identify an expansive process, and only an area of slightly high signal intensity close to the stenosed biliary ducts is present, detectable on T2w images. This is often difficult to differentiate from a benign infiltration, such as in sclerosing cholangitis and iatrogenic stenosis. In a case that we studied, recently treated by cholecystectomy, the neoplatic lesion was not clearly evident, and the stenosis was interpreted as an iatrogenic lesion. In these uncertain cases it is not even possible to a certain diagnosis of the tumor at pathological or bioptic (by brushing) evaluation.

Expansive forms with most evident aspect are appreciated especially at the hilar level, with a high signal intensity on T2w images and low signal intensity area on T1w images, located close to the portal vein, in correspondence to the biliary occlusion. Intrahepatic forms are often difficult to differentiate from the metastatic lesions. They present as solid tumors slightly with high signal intensity on T2w, with intrahepatic growth. In these cases the presence of biliary ducts' segmental dilatation cranially can lead to the correct preoperatory diagnosis, which must be confirmed by a percutaneous biopsy [4].

## Gallbladder Carcinoma

Gallbladder carcinoma is a rare neoplasm, but it is frequent among gastrointestinal neoplasms. It affects mostly women (4:1) aged 60–70 years. The correlation with cholelithiasis is very important (in 65%–95% of tumors) and is considered a predisposing factor, together with the associated chronic cholecystitis.

The most frequent symptom is jaundice due to biliary system infiltration at the cystic duct level or compression from subhilar lymphoadenopathies. However, the symptoms are very often weak and can correspond to those of cholelithiasis. Only ultrasound can generally detect the tumor associated with the stone. Finally, it is important to remember that in some cases the diagnosis of gallbladder carcinoma is reached only after cholecystectomy in stones associated with chronic cholecystitis; the pathological evaluation of the removed gallbladder allows identification of initial lesions (carcinoma in situ).

The prognosis of gallbladder carcinoma is poor, with survival to 6 months or, rarely, to 1 year. In most cases the therapy is only palliative to cure the jaundice.

In relation to the neoplastic growth type, it is possible to distinguish scirrhous forms, with galladder infiltration and organ complete disappearance, and papillar forms, where it is always possible to distinguish the cholecystic morphology, and the lesion has intraluminal growth. In all cases the hepatic infiltration at the gallbladder bed occurs very early, typically at the level of segment IV. Subhilar hepatic lymph nodes are also involved at a very early stage.

## MR Cholangiography

Jaundice and biliary obstruction are not present in all cases of gallbladder carcinoma. If they do occur, the level of the obstruction demonstrated on MR cholangiography corresponds to the site of the cystic duct outlet, with demonstration of the biliary ducts dilatated upstream and the regular size downstream.

The cystic duct is not evident owing to the neoplastic infiltration. In the larger forms a greater infiltration is present, up to the subhilar hepatic level. The same pattern can occur due to a wide (extensive) lymphoadenopathy, with stenosis of biliary system at the subhilar level. In both cases the biliary dilatation aspect is similar to that observed in the primary neoplastic lesion of the biliary system. The diagnosis is reached by means of the morphological MR conventional images evaluation (Fig. 8). If biliary infiltration and jaundice are not present, the biliary system appears with regular size on MR cholangiography. Theoretically, in the forms with intraluminar papillar growing the dilated gallbladder can be demonstrated, with the filling defect due to the neoplasm, as occurs in the invasive modalities using contrast media (ERCP and transhepatic cholangiography).

## MR Conventional Images

As noted above, MR conventional images allow the diagnosis of gallbladder carcinoma with high accuracy thanks to the presence of typical morphological aspects for this neoplastic forms [23]. The neoplasm is evident with a low signal intensity area on T1w images and a slightly high intensity area on T2w images at the level of gallbladder's bed. In the diffusely infiltrating forms the lesion can completely replace the gallbladder, which is no longer detectable. In the initial forms there is an irregular and segmental thickening of the gallbladder wall, with possible direct infiltration by contiguity of the adjacent hepatic parenchyma, at the level of segment IV. Instead in the polypoid forms an intraluminal expansive form is detected, with patent lumen of the gallbladder.

Evaluation of the presence of stone is very important since they are often associated with neoplasm. On MR stones are better detectable on T2-weighted images, with marked hypointensity (absence of free protons), which contrasts with the slightly high signal intensity area of the tumor. Finally, neoplastic extension along the cystic duct with subhilar hepatic involvement is often present, and lymphoadenopathies can be demonstrated. In the most advanced forms the hepatic involvement extends not only into segment IV,

**Fig. 8 a–e.** Carcinoma of the gallbladder involving the CBD. **a,b** CT images showing the thickened gallbladder wall (**a**) and the tissue surrounding the CBD (**b**).
**c** Axial T1-weighted image demonstrating the thickened gallbladder wall. **d** MRCP shows the obstruction at the level of the middle third of the CBD. **e** ERCP confirming MRCP findings

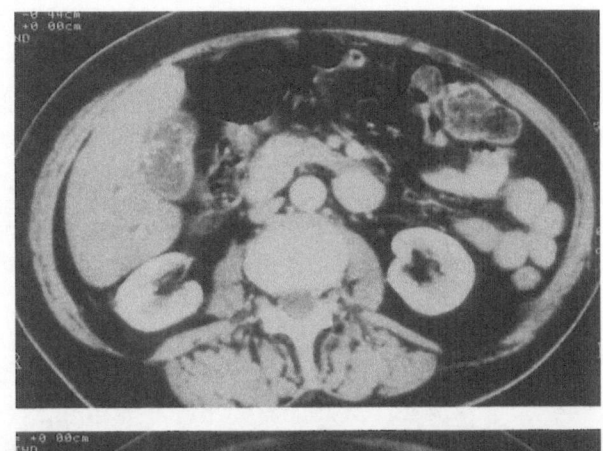

a

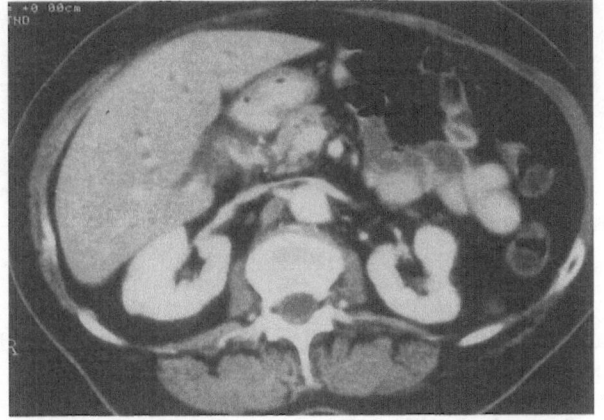

b

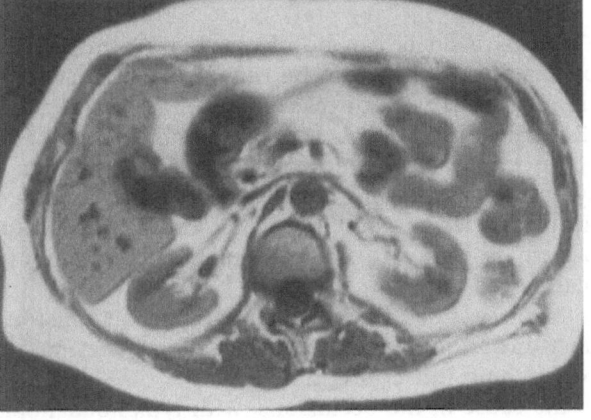

c

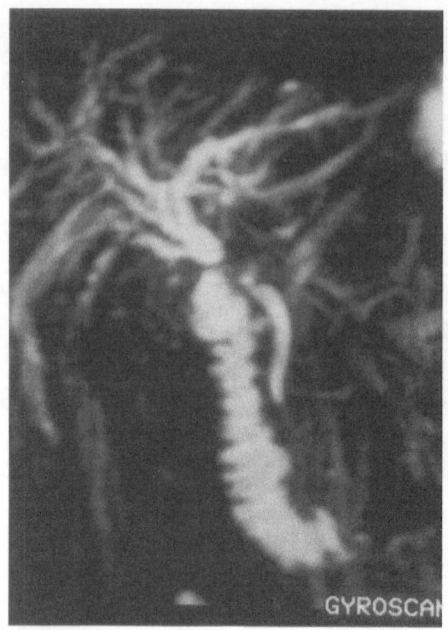 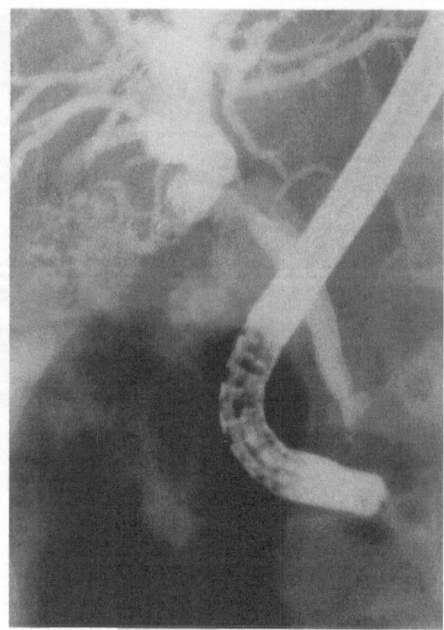

d                                                                                    e

**Fig. 8** (cont.)

and the diffusion to other organs must be evaluated. Recently we observed a cerebral metastasis several months after operation.

## Secondary Biliary Involvement

The biliary ducts can be obstructed by processes of other nature. The secondary involvement can be caused by subhilar lymphoadenopathies or hepatic metastasis with diffuse occlusion of segmental or subsegmental branches [24]. Hilar or subhilar hepatic lymphoadenopathy (Fig. 9) can cause an obstacle to the biliary flow and jaundice, and thus it can present itself with symptoms indistinguishable from those of lesions described above. Intestinal neoplastic lesions are those that cause hilar lymphnodal involvement. This pattern is therefore detected in the follow-up of colon and stomach neoplasms.

In these cases MR cholangiography demonstrates the intrahepatic biliary duct dilatation and the occlusion's hilar site. As for the other expansive processes, only MR conventional images (T1- and T2-weighted) allow detection of the cause of the occlusions, with lymphoadenopathy demonstration.

Multiple hepatic metastases can cause jaundice by two mechanism by a diffuse parenchymal metastatization, in absence of the main biliary system dilatation, or by a direct involvement of the biliary ducts at the segmental and subsegmental level.

**Fig. 9a–c.** Subhilar lymphadenopathy. **a, b** MR conventional images show the presence of multiple lymph
nodes at the hepatic hilum,
with involvement of portoca-
val nodes and peripancreatic
nodes. **c** MRCP shows the
presence of a smooth ex-
strinsic compression on the
CBD, with dilatation of the
bile ducts. The patient was
operated on and a diffuse
lymphadenopathy due to in-
differentiated carcinoma was
found

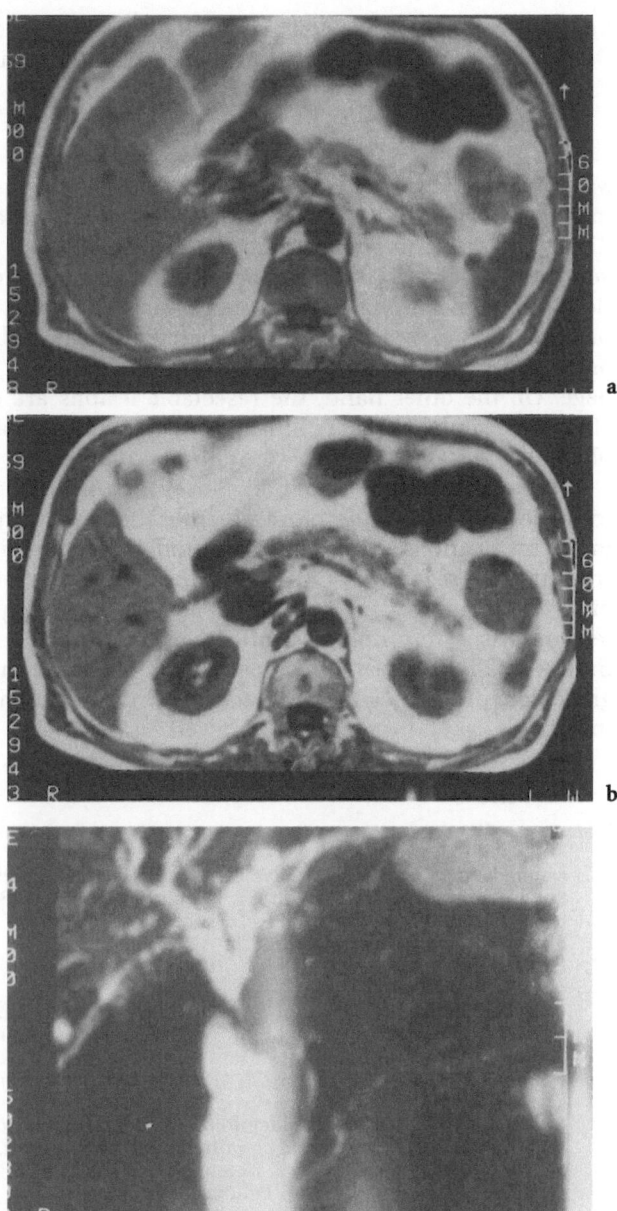

The simple diagnosis of multiple hepatic metastases by ultrasound would
not require the use of other diagnostic modalities. However, we are sure that
MR cholangiography can find a role in these cases, helping to demonstrate
the morphology of biliary involvement. The presence of dilated ducts, which
do not communicate with each other, could lead to interrupting every trans-

hepatic drainage attempt. This could reduce the useless and often injurious therapeutic procedures often performed in these patients.

## Conclusions

MR cholangiography has a clear role in evaluating neoplastic biliary involvement. In our study we have established that it can take completely the ERCP diagnostic role, supplying greater information. It is not limited to biliary involvement evaluation but defines the neoplasm extent through the association with conventional MR images, which allow the staging of the neoplastic process. In this way ERCP and percutaneous cholangiography are limited only to unresectable cases where it is necessary a jaundice palliative drainage. On the other hand, the resectable lesions are operated on immediately after the evaluation of the biliary involvement extension by MR cholangiography and the staging by MR conventional images.

MR sensitivity and specificity in evaluating malignant lesions are similar to those of CT. It is therefore possible that this technique can replace CT in many applications, becoming a second level modality, immediately after ultrasound. As regards to CT, in fact, the superiority of MR is due to the possibility of demonstrating the biliary tree morphology, over the neoplasm extension. Also, morphological MR images can be superior to CT images in defining small pancreatic lesions. Small lesions, which do not deform the glandular profile, can be detected with higher intrinsic contrast on MR images.

## References

1.  Robbins SL, Cotran R, Kumar V (1987) Pathological basis of diseases. Piccin, Padua
2.  Dooms GC, Hricak H, Crooks LE et al (1984) Magnetic resonance imaging of the limph nodes: comparison with CT. Radiology 153 719–728
3.  Steiner E, Stark DD, Hahn PF, Ferrucci JT et al (1984) "Imaging of pancreatic neoplasms: comparison of MR and CT. AJR 152:487
4.  Hamrick-Turner J, Abbitt PL, Ros PR (1992) Intrahepatic Cholangiocarcinoma: MR appearance. AJR 158:77–79
5.  Wallner BK, Schumacher KA, Weidenmainer W et al (1991) Dilated biliary tract: evaluation with MR cholangiography with T2-weighted contrast-enhanced fast sequence Radiology 181:805–808
6.  Higgins CB, Hricak H, Helms CA (1992) Magnetic Resonance of the body. Raven, New York
7.  Gordis L, Gold EB (1984) Epidemiology of pancreatic cancer. World J Surg 8:808–821
8.  Sarner M (1986) Pancreatitis: definition and classification. The exocrine pancreas: biology, pathobiology and disease. Raven, New York, pp 459–464
9.  Schultz RE, Finkler NJ (1980) Pancreatic calcification and pancreatic carcinoma: the relationship reconsidered. Mt Sinai J Med 47:622–626
10. Smith W, Reid A, Hutchinson JMS et al (1982) NMR imaging of the pancreas. Radiology 165 677–680
11. Tscholakoff D, Hricak H, Thoeni R et al (1987) MR imaging in the diagnosis of pancreatic disease. AJR 149 (2):703–709
12. Anacker H, Weiss HD, Kramann B (1977) ERCP in diseases of the biliary tract. In endoscopic retrograde pancreticocholangiography (ERCP). Springer, Berlin Heidelberg New York
13. Muller MF, Meyenberger C, Bertschinger P et al (1994) Pancreatic tumors: evaluation with endoscopic US, CT and MR imaging. Radiology 190:745–751

14. Tscholakoff D, Hricak H, Thoeni R et al (1987) MR imaging in the diagnosis of pancreatic diseases. AJR 148 703–709
15. Kenney PJ, Morgan DE, Rominger MB et al (1992) Advanced MR imaging of the pancreas. Radiology 185 (P) 391
16. Kraus BB, Ros PR (1994) Insulinoma: diagnosis with fat-suppressed MR imaging. AJR 162:69–70
17. Mitchell DG, Vinitsky S, Saponaro S et al (1991) Liver and pancreas: improved spin-echo T1 contrast by shorter echo time and fat suppression at 1.5T. Radiology 178:67–71
18. Mitchell DG, Shapiro M, Schuricht A et al (1992) Pancreatic disease: findings on state of the art MR images. AJR 159:533–538
19. Chezmar JL, Rumancik WM, Megibow AJ et al (1988) Liver and abdominal screening in patient with cancer: CT versus MR imaging. Radiology 168:43–47
20. Dillon E, Peel AL, Perkin GJ (1981) The diagnosis of primary bile duct carcinoma (cholangiocarcinoma) in the jaundiced patient. Clin Radiol 132:311
21. Dooms GC, Kerlan RK Jr, Hricak H et al (1986) Cholangiocarcinoma: imaging by MR. Radiology 159:89–94
22. Montana MA, Rohrmann CA (1986) Cholangiocarcinoma in a choledocal cyst: preoperative diagnosis. AJR 147:516–517
23. Brink JA, Borrello JA (1995) MR imaging of the biliary system. Magn Reson Imaging Clin N Am 3(1):143–60
24. Soyer P, Laissy JP, Bluemke DA, Sibert A, Menu Y (1995) Bile duct involvement in hepatocellular carcinoma: MR demonstration. Abdom Imaging 20(2):118–21

# CHAPTER 8

# MR Pancreatography

## Introduction

MRCP is a valuable technique for representating the pancreatic ducts. More important than for detecting the biliary ducts and fundamental for visualizating the pancreatic duct is its dilatation, even if minimal [1]. Under normal conditions the pancreatic duct diameter ranges between 2 and 3 mm [2, 3]. The presence of accessory pancreatic ducts is a frequent finding; in particular glandular pathologies may be selectively dilated.

### Anatomy

The pancreatic duct has a diameter of about 2 mm, with a course along the entire length of the gland [4]. It is reached perpendicularly by small ducts arising from the lobules [5, 6]. In about 80% of cases it joins the main biliary duct at the level of the papilla of Vater, while in the remaining cases it enters the duodenum in its proximity [7, 8]. It also often exists an accessory pancreatic duct entering the duodenum above the papilla (Figs. 1, 2). In a small percentage of cases the accessory duct is absent and is often only a collateral duct [9–13].

MRCP allows good visualization of the normal pancreatic duct. In a study by Soto et al. [14] the specificity of MRCP in demonstrating normal pancreatic ducts was 69%. On the other hand, when single slices were examined, the specificity increased to 81%.

### Semeiotics

Any of several pathologies, most often arising from the pancreas itself, may cause dilatation of the pancreatic duct. A pancreatic duct system dilatation can be caused by inflammatory processes, either acute or chronic, more often by neoplastic masses [15–17].

MRCP semeiotics is very similar to that of ERCP, although many differences exist between the two methods [18, 19]. Main and secondary pancreatic duct morphology may often lead to a correct diagnosis. In particular there exist some semeiological criteria for the diagnosis of pancreatic carcinoma, among which are a pancreatic duct and sometimes also CBD stenosis with rigid and irregular profiles, with associated uniform dilatation above the stenosis itself (Fig. 3).

On the other hand, the criteria for diagnosis of chronic pancreatitis are an irregular dilatation of secondary ducts, alternating stenoses and dilatations of

**Fig. 1. a** MIP-reconstructed image shows dilation of both the main pancreatic duct and the accessory duct. **b** A better evaluation of the accessory duct is possible on source image

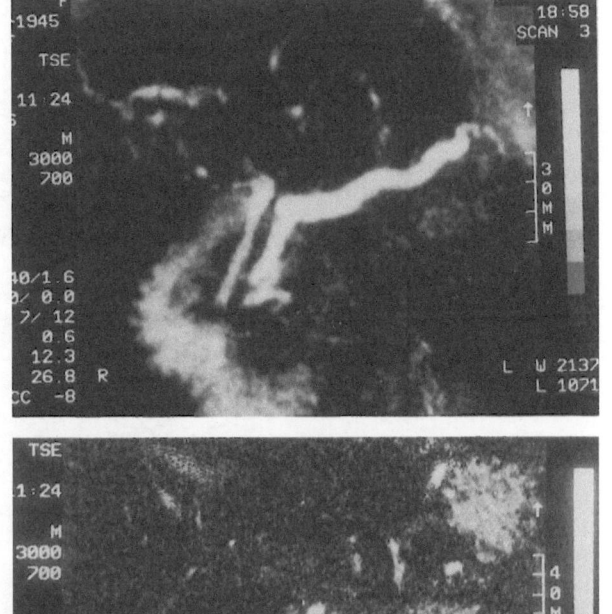

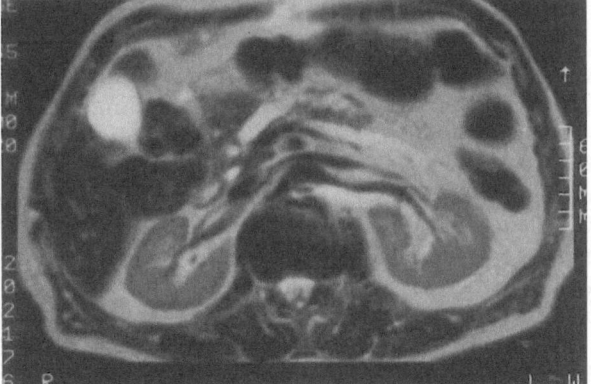

**Fig. 2 a–c.** Chronic pancreatitis. **a** The axial T2-weighted image shows diffuse signal alterations of the pancreas with wide dilation of the Wirsung duct. **b** MRCP show dilation of the Wirsung duct and dilation of the accessory duct. **c** The source image provides a better delineation of dilated secondary ducts

**Fig. 2** (cont.)

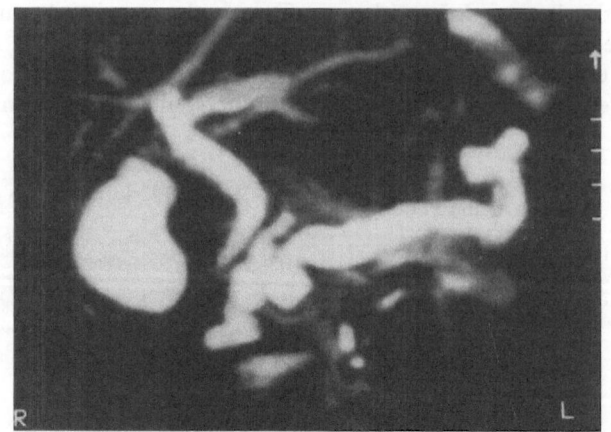

b

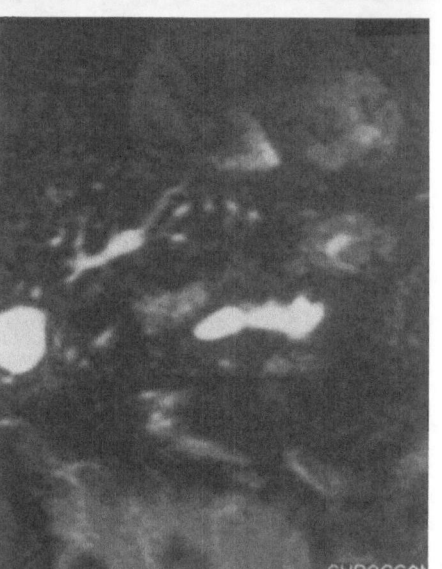

c

the Wirsung duct (beaded appearance), and a smooth progressive stenosis (Figs. 4, 5). One of the more frequent findings at pancreatography is the presence of filling defects within the pancreatic duct, which may be due to the presence of stones (Figs. 5, 6). Their presence is easily recognized on MRCP. They all appear as areas of signal void within the pancreatic duct lumen. On ERCP it is often possible to detect the presence of calcifications, mucin, and small soft tissue masses and therefore to recognize their nature. The role of MRCP can be the identificaton of the filling defects, with ERCP performed for stone removal, whatever their content.

Another frequent finding are cystic masses (Figs. 7–9). On both MRI and MRCP the presence of fluid within the cyst constitutes a natural contrast,

**Fig. 3.** Pancreatic carcinoma, where the obstruction of the pancreatic duct is associated with CBD stenosis and uniform dilatation above the stenosis itself

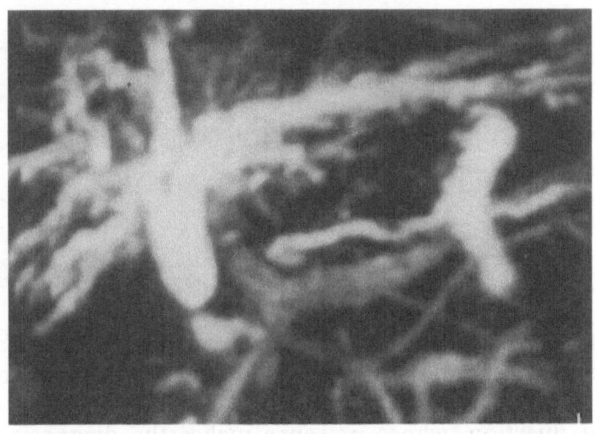

**Fig. 4 a–c.** Diffuse chronic pancreatitis. **a** Axial T2-weighted image showing multiple cystic lesions in the head of the pancreas associated with diffuse signal intensity alterations. **b** MIP-reconstructed MRCP image depicts the "beaded" appearance of the Wirsung duct and the dilation of the CBD. **c** Magnification of the Wirsung duct better depicting the typical findings of chronic pancreatitis

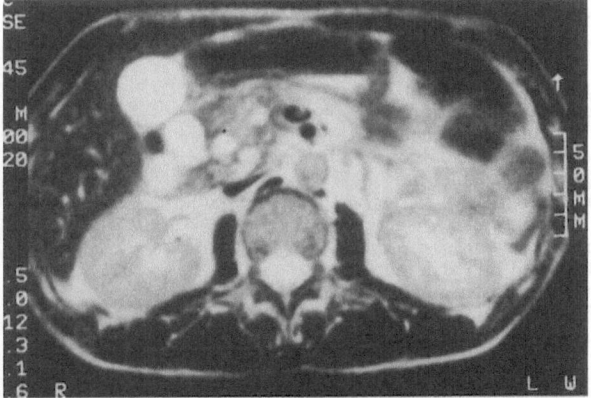

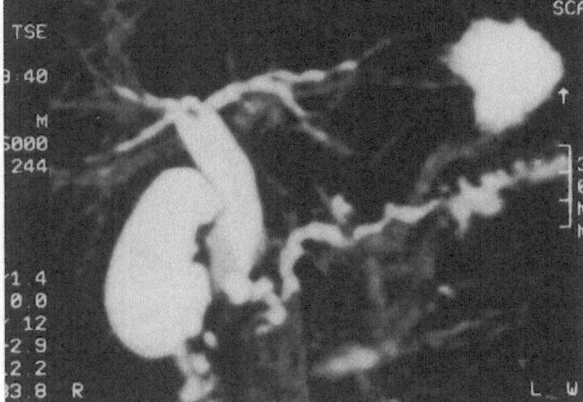

**Fig. 4** (cont.)

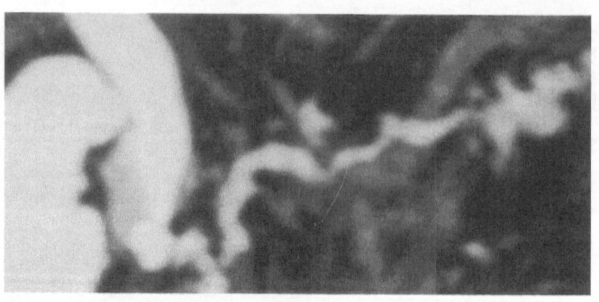

c

making their identification easy. Fundamental for correct treatment planning is confirmation of communication between the cyst and the pancreatic ducts. On MRCP this is not possible because of the absence of an intraluminal contrast injection, whose presence makes the diagnosis easy on ERCP. On the other hand, on MRCP, with the association of conventional MR images, the relationship of the cystic lesion with the glandular parenchyma and ductal system can be easily confirmed [20].

**Fig. 5. a** MRCP image of chronic pancreatitis with smooth progressive stenosis and irregular dilatation of secondary ducts, alternating stenoses and dilatations of the Wirsung duct (beaded appearance). **b,c** Source images better depict the smooth progressive stenosis and multiple filling defect identified as stones. **d** Axial T1-weighted image demonstrates the diffuse alteration of the pancreatic parenchyma as in chronic pancreatitis

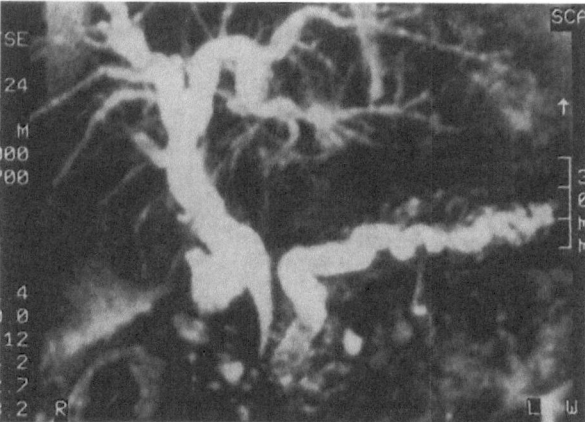

a

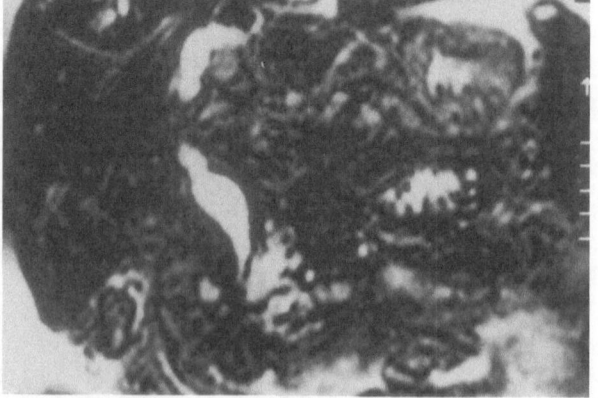

b

**Fig. 5.** (cont.)

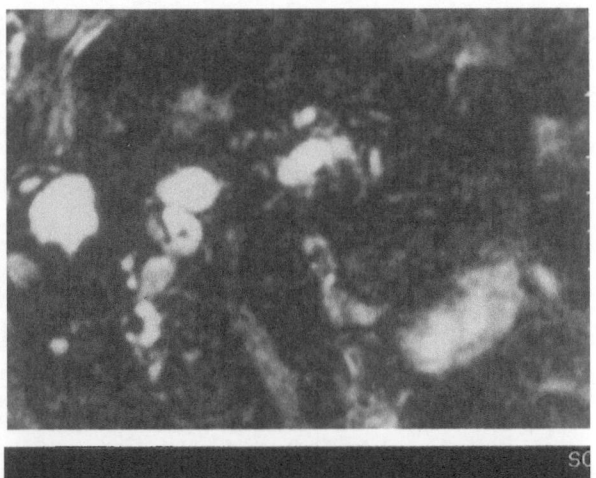

c

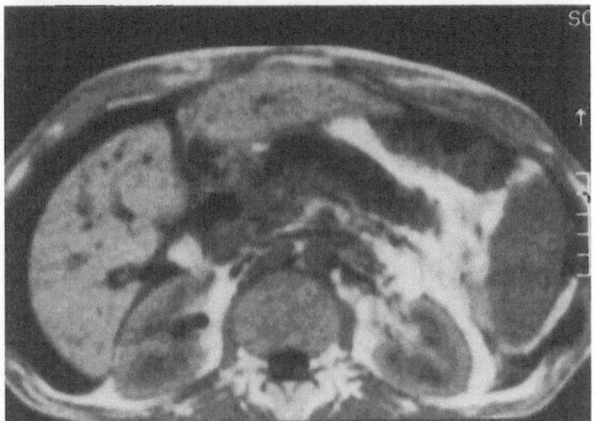

d

**Fig. 6. a** Axial T2-weighted image shows diffuse alterations of the pancreas. **b** On MRCP dilation of the Wirsung duct with multiple stenosis is clear. **c** On source image multiple filling defects are present

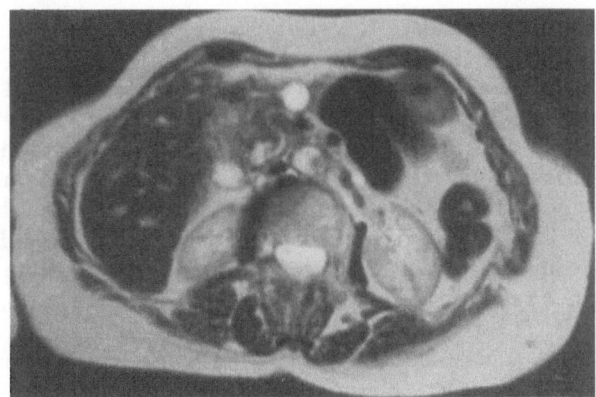

a

**Fig. 6.** (cont.)

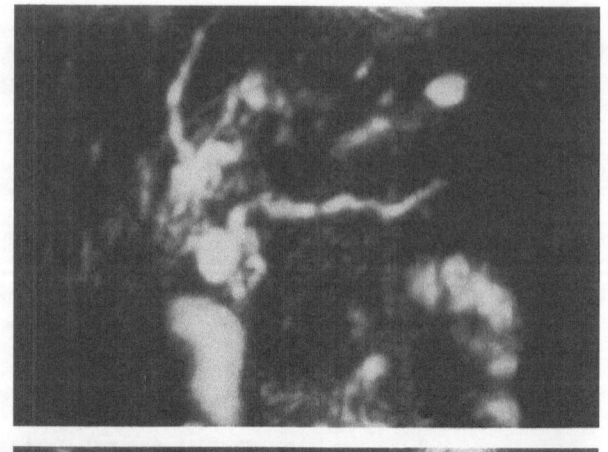

b

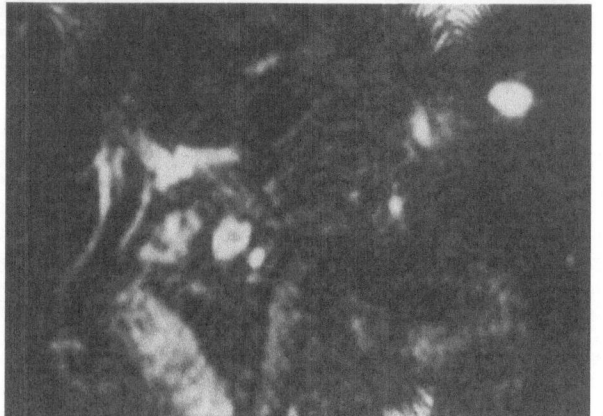

c

## Pathological Findings

### Acute Pancreatitis

Acute pancreatitis may be caused by any of several different causes, most commonly biliary lithiasis and alcohol abuse, Their differentiation can be clinically difficult, making necessary a pancreatography [21]. The mechanism for lithiasic pancreatitis is not known, although it might be caused by obstruction of the pancreatic duct. Particularly on the basis of this hypothesis ERCP has become particularly popular in the 1990s. Nevertheless the risk of procedure related complications is quite high, and the role of ERCP therefore has not yet been defined [22–25]. On the other hand, the possibility of having direct cholangiographic images noninvasively in cases of suspected lithiastic acute pancreatitis must be considered an important advance, especially for treatment planning.

**Fig. 7.** Pseudocyst of the tail of the pancreas. MRCP shows the contiguity between the dilated Wirsung duct and the pseudocyst

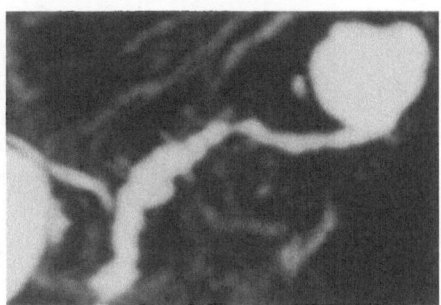

**Fig. 8.** a MRCP image of a lobulated pseudocyst of the tail of the pancreas. b The source image permits evaluating the inhomogeneous signal due to hematic content. c Also on axial T1-weighted image the pseudocyst can be easily evaluated

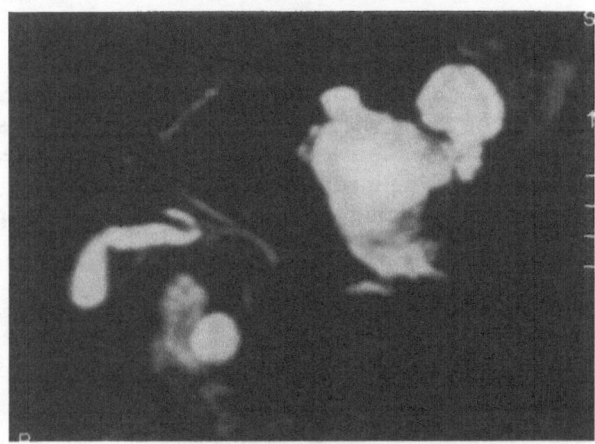

a

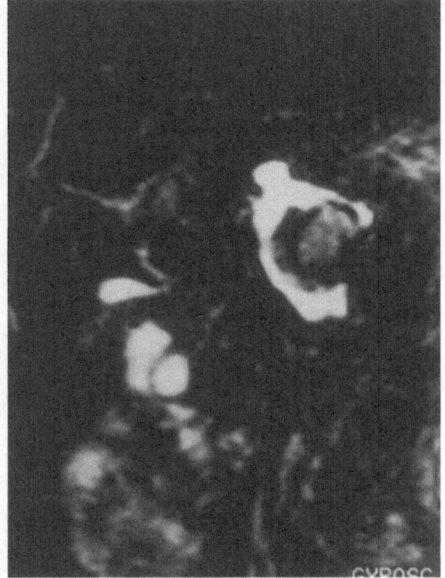

b

**Fig. 8.** (cont.)

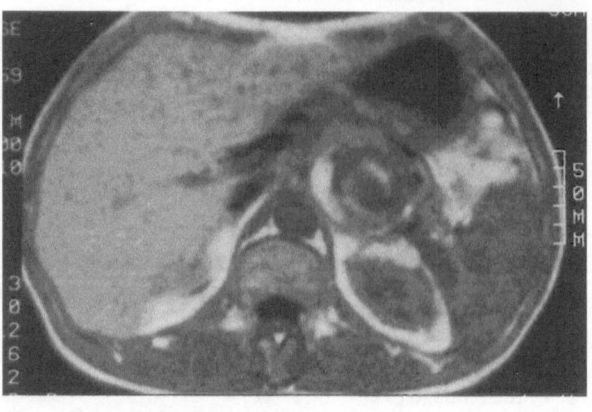

c

Similarly to the case of bile duct lithiasis, to increase the detection rate the analysis of single slices is fundamental, in which small filling defects are easily identifiable. The use of MRCP in acute pancreatitis due to suspected lithiasis is not yet defined; nevertheless the technique can be proposed in all cases in which a diagnostic direct cholangio-pancretogram is required. Wide

**Fig. 9 a–c.** Pseudocyst of the head of the pancreas. T1-weighted (a) and T2-weighted (b) images demonstrate an enlargement of the head of the pancreas with multiple pseudocysts. c On MRCP the pseudocysts are well depicted and seem not to be in communication with the Wirsung duct

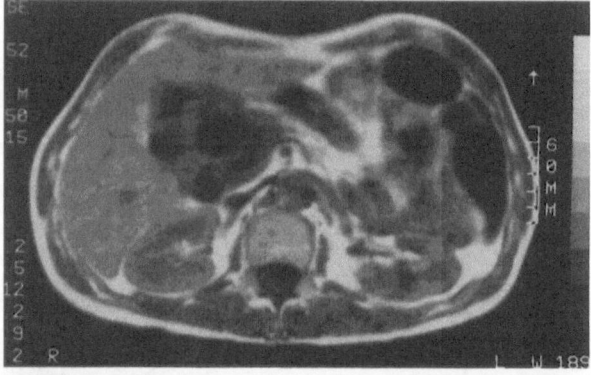

a

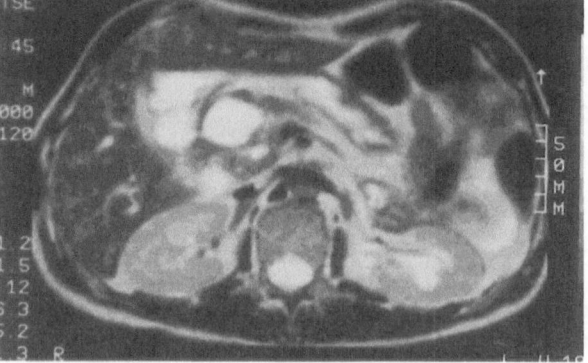

b

**Fig. 9.** (cont.)

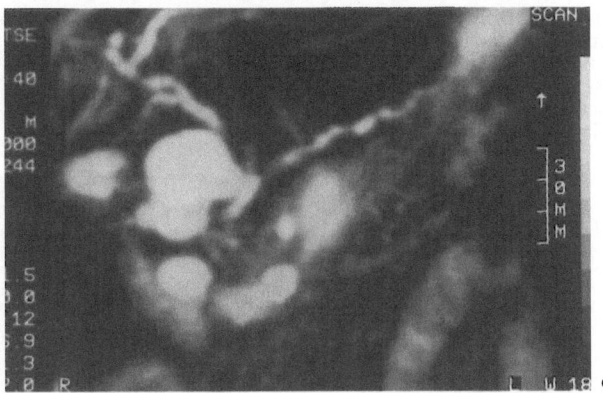

c

clinical randomized trials should be performed to verify the value of MRCP in acute pancreatitis.

### Chronic Pancreatitis

The diagnosis of chronic pancreatitis is very difficult in many instances, especially because of the poor correlation between symptoms and the morphological features seen at diagnostic examinations.

Retrograde pancreatography is often necessary whenever noninvasive diagnostic examinations are not clearly indicative in patients with abdominal pain, probably of pancreatic origin. Nevertheless, in some cases even retrograde pancreatography cannot provide sufficient information for a correct diagnosis. For this purpose and to examine the pancreatic parenchyma together with the ductal system, endoscopic ultrasound has been proposed, but with results that are not yet completely satisfactory.

In MR the possibility of combining cholangiographic with conventional images may be advantageous for the study of chronic pancreatitis. MRCP images now allow detection of pancreatic duct dilatations and stenoses even at the level of peripheral branches, where modifications are often seen in early chronic pancreatitis changes (Figs. 10, 11). The fine details evident with ERCP cannot be seen with MRCP. This depends mainly upon the different condition of the pancreatic system during the two examinations. During retrograde pancreatography contrast medium injection creates a high-pressure condition with consequent further dilatation of the ducts. At the same time MRCP reflects the natural state of the ducts, similarly to what is seen on ERCP after the cessation of contrast injection.

Chronic pancreatitis in advanced cases can be easily diagnosed by both CT and ultrasound, while the identification of initial slight alterations of pancreatic ducts requires the ERCP [26]. The retrograde filling of the ducts allows detection of the irregular dilatations of lateral branches and of wall irregularities of the main pancreatic duct. One of the main features of moderate and severe chronic pancreatitis is the stenosis of the main duct, generally as-

**Fig. 10 a,b.** Diffuse chronic pancreatitis. **a** MIP-reconstructed image shows a diffuse dilation of the Wirsung duct. **b** On source image dilation of secondary ducts can be appreciated

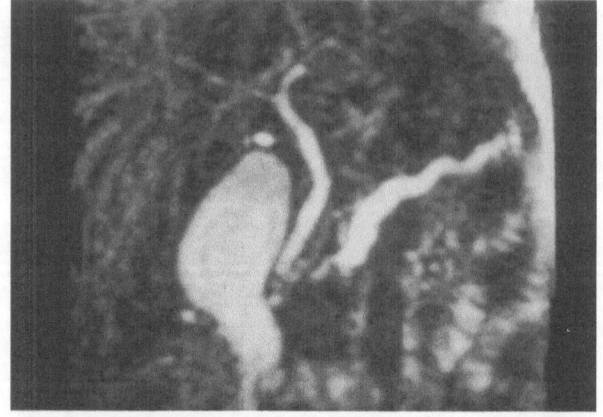

a

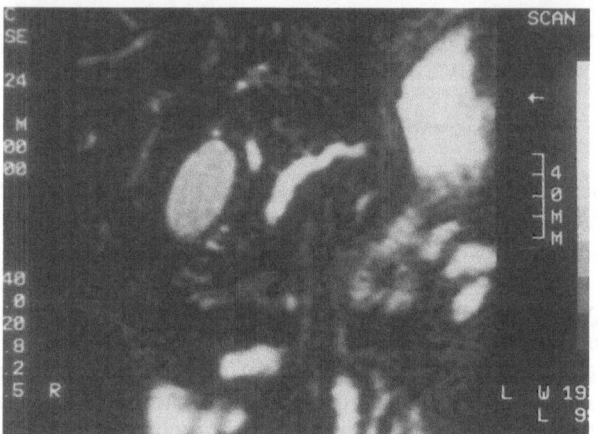

b

sociated with irregular dilatations; their combination constitutes the typical pattern of the beaded appearance. Another frequent finding of chronic pancreatitis is the presence of stones, which on ERCP are seen as filling defects, while on MRCP as areas of signal void. The sensitivity of MRCP in the detection of pancreatic stones is quite high. Takehara et al. [27] have reported sensitivity in the detection of filling defects between 92% and 100% depending on the location of the stones (tail 92%, head and body 100%). Detectability, which can be improved by examination of single slices, is highly dependent on filling defects size. In the series of Soto et al. [14, 28], the sensitivity for detecting pancreatic duct dilatation was 87%–100%; strictures were detected in 75% of cases, with a single false-positive finding; in the two patients with small intraluminal stones they were always identified.

Particularly in the evaluation of patients with chronic pancreatitis MRCP may become a very useful method, especially considering the high risk associated with ERCP.

**Fig. 11 a,b.** Diffuse chronic pancreatitis. **a** MRCP image shows a tortuous and dilated Wirsung duct. **b** Axial T1-weighted image depicting the diffuse alteration of the pancreatic parenchyma

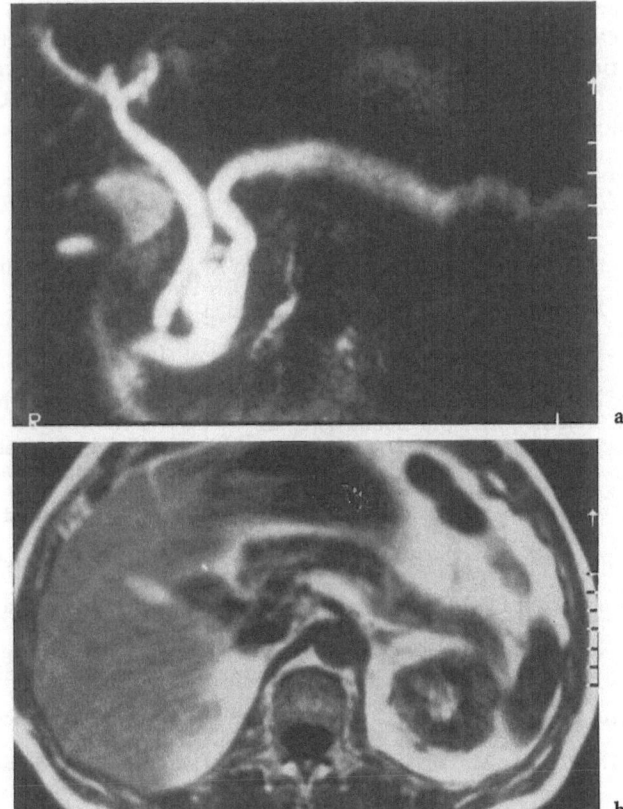

## Pancreatic Cancer

Evaluating dilatation of the pancreatic duct in pancreatic cancer is easy with MRCP. In addition to showing the biliary dilatation, MRCP provides consistent images of the dilated duct, with a resolution only slightly lower than that of ERCP. Moreover, MRCP images are compared to conventional MR images, with a complete examination of the bile ducts, pancreatic duct, and pancreatic parenchyma, which allows the definition and staging of the tumor (see Chap. 7) [29, 30].

## Differential Diagnosis

The appearance of the pancreatic duct may have an important role in defining the underlining pathology, either phlogistic or neoplastic. Although this is true in typical cases, with irregular dilatation or beaded appearance in pancreatitis, or with smooth uniform dilatation in case of cancer, there are many instances when the data of MRCP cannot provide the correct diagnosis. This means that focal chronic pancreatitis may resemble cancer, while cancer rarely simulate the inflammatory disease. In the presence of calcification MR may lack the high specificity of CT. However, the evidence of areas of very low signal intensity suggests the presence of calcified areas, indicative for phlogistic disease.

## References

1. BolondiL, Gaiani S, Gullo L, Labo' G (1984) Secretin administration induces a dilatation of main pancreatic duct. Dig Dis Sci 29:802–808
2. Moore KL (1985) Clinically oriented anatomy. Williams and Wilkins, Baltimore, pp 220–224
3. Lawson TL, Berland LL, Foley WD et al (1982) Ultrasonic visualization of the pancreatic duct. Radiology 144:865–871
4. Hadidi A (1983) Pancreatic duct diameter: sonographic measurement in normal subjects. J Clin Ultrasound 11:17–22
5. Donovan PJ (1983) Technique of examination and normal pancreatic anatomy. In Siegelman SS (ed) Computed tomography of the pancreas, Churchill Livingston, New York, pp 1–32
6. Lawson TL, Berland LL, Foley WD et al (1982) Ultrasound visualization of the pancreatic duct. Radiology 144:865–871
7. Parulekar SG (1980) Ultrasonic evaluation of the pancreatic duct. J Clin Ultrasound 8:457–463
8. Bryan PJ (1982) Appearance of normal pancreatic duct: a study using real-time ultrasound. J Clin Ultrasound 10:63–66
9. Schulte SJ (1994) Embryology, normal variation and congenital anomalies of the pancreas. In: Margulis and Burhenne's alimentary tract radiology. Mosby, St. Louis, pp 1039–1051
10. Agha FD, Williams KD, (1987) Pancreas divisum: incidence, detection, and clinical significance. Am J Gastroenterol 82:315–320
11. Delhaye M, Engelholm L, Cremer M (1985) Pancreas divisum: congenital anatomy variant or anomaly: contribution of endoscopiy retrograde dorsal pancreatography. Gastroenterology 89:951–958
12. Delhaye M, Engelholm L, Cremer M (1988) Pancreas divisum: controvetrsial clinical significance. Dig Dis 6:30–39
13. Cotton PB (1980) Congenital anomaly of pancreas divisum as a cause of obstuctive pain and pancreatitis. Gut 21:105–114
14. Soto JA, Barish MA, Yucel EK et al (1995) Pancreatic duct: MR cholangiopancreatography with a three-dimensional fast spin-echo technique
15. Schneck CD (1983) The anatomical basis of abdominopelvic sectional imaging.In: Joseph HEA, Cosgrove DO (eds) Ultrasound in inflammatory disease. Clin Diagn Ultrasound 11:13–41
16. Callen PW, London SS, Moss AA (1980) Computed tomographic evaluation of the dilated pancreatic duct: the value of thinsection collimation. Radiology 134:253–255
17. Callen PW, London SS, Moss AA (1980) Computed tomohgraphic evaluation of the dilated pancreatic duct: the value of thinsection collimation. Radiology 134:253–255
18. Walner BK, Schumcker KA, Weidenmaier W, Freidrich JM (1991) Dilated biliary tract: evaluation with MR cholangiography with a heavily T2-weighted contrast-enhanced fast sequence. Radiology 181:805–808
19. Soto JA, Yucel EK, Barish MA, Chuttani R, Ferrucci JT (1994) MR cholangiopancreatography: correlation with endoscopic retrograde cholangiopancreatography (abstr). Radiology 193:133
20. Outwater EK, Gordon SJ (1994) Imaging the pancreatic and biliary ducts with MR. Radiology 192:19–21
21. Hamilton I, Lintott DJ, Rothwell J, Axon ATR (1983) Acute pancreatitis following endoscopic retrograde cholangiopancreatography. Clin Radiol 34:543–546
22. Thoeni RF, Fel SC, Goldberg HI (1990) CT detection of asymptomatic pancreatitis following ERCP. Gastrointest Radiol 15:291–295
23. Shimizu S, Tada M, Kawai K (1992) Diagnostic ERCP. Endoscopy 24:95–99

24. Hamilton I, Lintott DJ, Rothwell J, Axon ATR (1983) Acute pancreatitis following endoscopic retrograde cholangiopancreatography. Clin Radiol 34:543–546
25. Bilbao MK, Dotter CT, Lee TG, Katon RM (1976) Complications of endoscopic retrograde cholangiopancreatography (ERCP): a study of 10,000 cases. Gastroenterology 70:314–320
26. Axon A (1989) Endoscopic retrograde cholangiopancreatography in chronic pancreatitis: Cambridge classification. Radiol Clin North Am 27:39–50
27. Takehara Y, Ichijo K, Tooyama N et al (1994) Breath-hold MR cholangiopancreatography with a long-echo train fast spin-echo sequence and a surface coil in chronic pancreatitis. Radiology 192:73–78
28. Barish MA, Yucel EK, Soto JA, Chuttani R, Ferrucci JT (1995) MR cholangiopancreatography: efficacy of three-dimensional turbo, spin-echo technique. AJR 165:295–300
29. Outwater EK, Gordon SJ (1994) Imaging the pancreatic and biliary ducts with MR. Radiology 192:19–21
30. Barish MA, Soto JA, Shah J, Silver MS, Ferrucci JT, Yucel EK (1994) 3D multislab turbo spin echo: a novel technique for MR cholangiography (abstract). In: Proceedings of the Society of Magnetic Resonance, Berkeley, p297

# CHAPTER 9

# Biliary-Enteric Anastomoses

## Introduction

Indications for surgical creation of biliary-enteric anastomosis (BEA) have been significantly reduced by improvements of interventional endoscopy (sphincterotomy and biliary endoprosthesis placement), especially in patients with malignant obstructions and choledocholithiasis. However, surgery is still indicated when the CBD is larger than 1.5 cm, when large stones occupy the CBD, and when tight and extensive stenosis of the papilla are present, especially in the long-term treatment of elderly patients. Selecting the intestinal segment to use in performing BEA is still controversial and seems to depend on the experience of the surgeon rather than on any really objective criteria. The indications for performing BEA include Mirizzi's syndrome (0.5%–2% of choledocholithiasis [1]) and benign stenosis of the CBD due to iatrogenic lesions. These have recently increased in number as a consequence of the greater use of laparoscopic cholecystectomy.

Bismuth has clearly demonstrated the different kinds of CBD stenosis due to fibrous tissue proliferation [2]. The morphology of these strictures can be summarized considering three lines, the first crossing the proximal and distal margins of the biliary carrefour and the third one 2 cm below the latter. In this way it is possible to differentiate lower (type 1), middle (type 2) and higher stenoses (type 3). In addition, another type of stenosis (type 4) is when the biliary carrefour is involved, and when an abnormality of the biliary carrefour is also present (type 5). In these cases surgical biliary drainage is performed by a large anastomosis using the biliary tracts free from fibrosis to prevent recurrency of the stenosis [3–7].

To visualize and study BEA correctly it is essential to know all the possible anastomoses generally performed in the majority of surgical centers, which vary in relation to the original type of stenosis. With low and middle stenosis (type 1 and 2) the anastomosis can be either choledochojejunal or hepaticojejunal, whereas with high stenosis (type 3) a Roux-en-Y anastomosis is mandatory. In type 4 stenosis surgery includes a first phase aimed at carrefour reconstruction, and if this is not possible the preparation of two different anastomosis between the biliary ducts and the jejunal loop. As consequence of the surgical therapeutic approach a duodenobiliary reflux occurs constantly in patients treated with choledochoduodenal anastomosis, and a bile flux diversion is present in hepaticojejunal anastomosis. Therefore angiocholitis and pancreatitis are quite frequent due to stenosis of the anastomosis or to stone migration, and they must be recognized by the radiologist in the study of patients treated with BEA [8–10].

Reasons for investigating the patency of biliary-enteric anastomosis and the anatomy of the bile ducts include fevers of uncertain etiology, suspected cholangitis, pancreatitis, right upper quadrant pain, abnormal liver function tests, and jaundice. The incidence of long-term complications (strictures, stones, cholangitis) following hepatico- or choledocho-jejunostomy for benign lesions has been reported as 7%–23% [9, 11, 12]. In particular, recurrence of stenosis is about 18% following first surgical intervention and is up to 26% following the second surgical treatment [13].

Proper study is very important, especially in patients treated for benign disease, who have a long life expectancy. These patients require long-term follow-up, and the presence of mild symptoms need a correct assessment of the biliary tree before planning any further treatment.

## Imaging Modalities

Methods commonly employed include, intravenous cholangiography, ultrasound, biliscintigraphy, CT, PTC, and ERCP. Intravenous cholangiogram is often useless and has a high rate of complications [14]. Ultrasound is undoubtly the technique of choice for initial evaluation of the bile ducts, particularly in patients with jaundice [15]. However, it is less useful in patients with surgically created biliary-enteric anastomoses because gas in the bile ducts may mimic ductal stones and create artifacts. According to some authors, the upright ultrasound examination is valuable in assessing the presence of air in the biliary ducts, which reveals the patency of the anastomosis or the presence of air-fluid levels and suggests a partial obstruction. The absence of air may indicate a stenosis [16]. CT findings are similar to those of ultrasound and have similar disadvantages [17]. Biliscintigraphy has an important role in assessing functional obstruction of the biliary tree. It can also be performed in patients with elevated serum bilirubin levels, but its main limitation is the lack of a morphological representation of the biliary tree [18].

ERCP has been used with diagnostic purposes in symptomatic patients treated with biliary-enteric anastomoses. However, its use is confined to patients with anastomosis not beyond the duodenum and without a prior gastro-jejunostomy. ERCP is difficult if not impossible in patients with anastomoses of bile duct to jejunal loops or Roux-en-Y loops. Complications such as stones, strictures, and fistulae can indeed be visualized via the retrograde injection of contrast material. It requires highly trained personnel and complex, expensive equipment [19].

PTC is undoubtedly valuable, but it is risky, expensive, and highly invasive. Its, diagnostic role may be limited as a preliminary step to interventional procedures, such as balloon dilation of the anastomosis and stone removal, as an alternative to surgical correction [20].

Although ERCP and PTC definitely play an important role in the evaluation of BEA, the high frequency of complications associated with them cannot be overlooked. The incidence of sepsis has been reported as 1.4% during PTC and 1.12% during ERCP, with death in 0.20% for PTC and 0.17% for ERCP [21].

## MRCP

Recently MRCP, a noninvasive, non-operator-dependent technique, has gained a relevant role in the evaluation of bile duct disease, with a great accuracy in evaluating bile duct obstruction, choledocholithiasis, and malignant obstructions [22–24].

In addition to an accurate visualization of the anastomosis, other radiological findings to be investigated with this imaging modality include the dilation of the bile ducts, the presence of stenosis at the level of the anastomosis, signs of cholangitis represented by bile ducts irregularity, and stones.

The main technical advantage over ERCP, other than invasiveness, is the possibility to be performed in patients undergoing a prior gastro-jejunostomy and in those with anastomosis beyond the duodenum (Figs. 1–4). MRCP allows a correct evaluation of the site of the anastomosis, and the cause of obstruction. The stenoses are better depicted if source images are also evaluated, especially concerning their morphology and extension (Figs. 5, 6). In a large number of cases MIP reconstruction overestimates the stenosis of the anastomosis, and the relationship between the anastomosis and the intestinal loop is missed. As is well illustrated in Chap. 5, stones are easily recognized as low-intensity structures surrounded by the high signal intensity of the bile [24]. However, in the case of 2–3 mm round-shaped, low signal intensity images, differential diagnosis between small stones and air bubbles is extremely difficult, but it is not clinically relevant. Of course, the evaluation of single slices is mandatory for the correct assessment both of anastomosis and of the presence of stones. On MIP-reconstructed images stones can be obscured by the high signal intensity of the surrounding bile (Fig. 7–9).

**Fig. 1.** A 70-year-old woman undergoing hepatico-jejunostomy. Normal appearance of the anastomosis (*arrowhead*) without dilation of the intrahepatic ducts

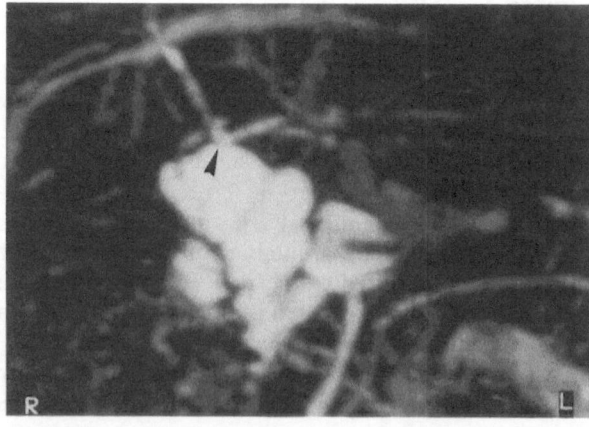

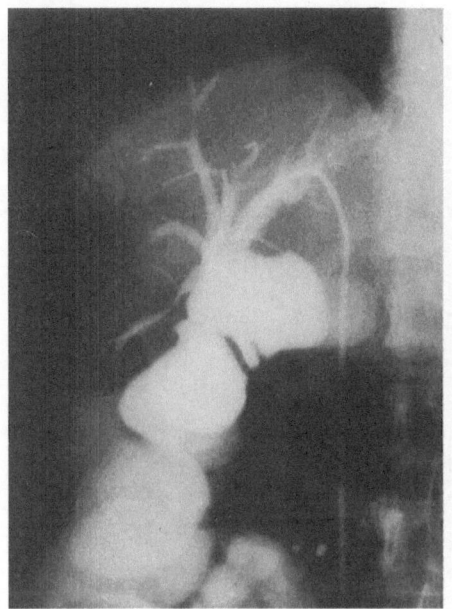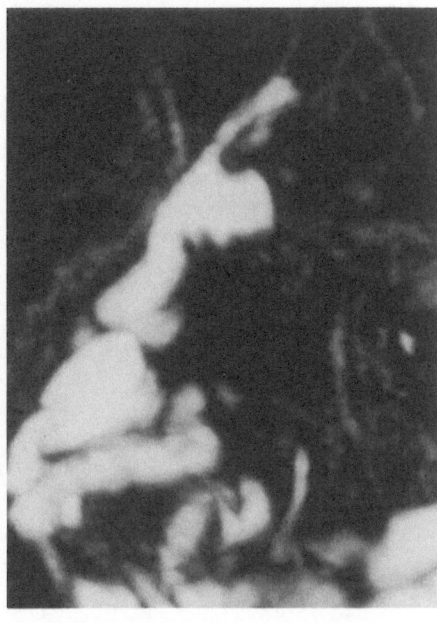

a                                                                         b

**Fig. 2 a,b.** A 58-year-old woman undergoing hepatico-jejunostomy. **a** PTC performed to dilate stenosis of the anastomosis demonstrates the anatomy of the hepatic ducts. **b** MRCP
performed after remotion of percutaneous drainage shows slight dilation of the left hepatic
duct and normal size of right hepatic duct

**Fig. 3.** A 61-year-old man
undergoing choledocho-duodenostomy. Normal appear-
ance of the anastomosis (*ar-
row*) with no dilation of the
bile ducts; the native CBD
can be observed

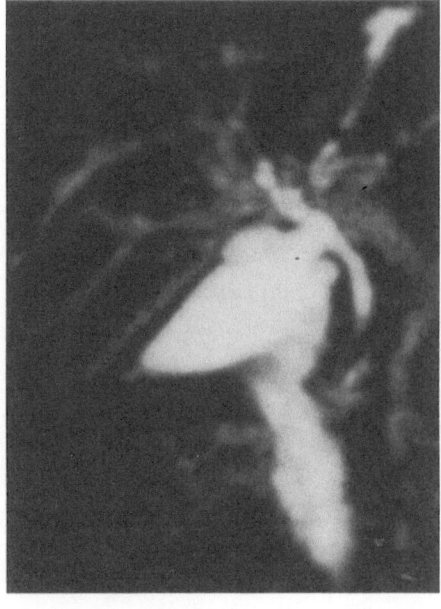

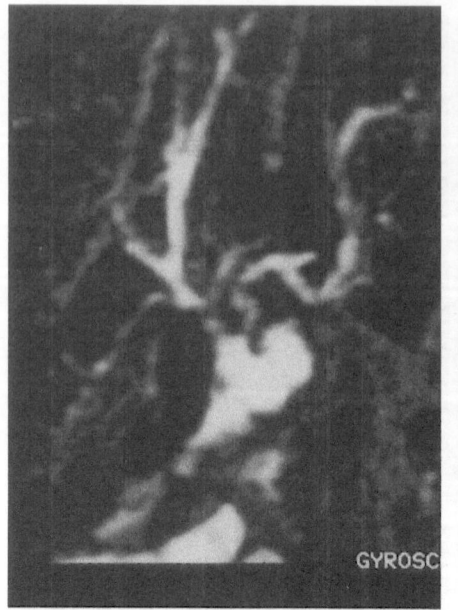
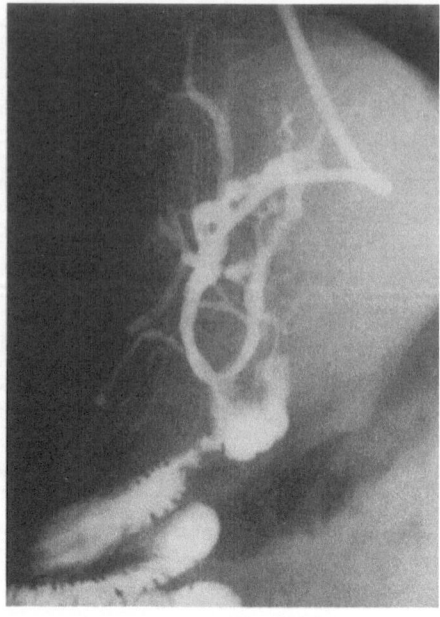

a                                                                                    b

**Fig. 4 a,b.** A 73-year-old man undergoing hepatico-jejunostomy. **a** MRCP shows a mild stenosis with dilation of the hepatic ducts. Minor signs of cholangitis are evident. **b** Five days after MRCP, diagnostic PTC confirms MR findings

**Fig. 5 a,b.** A 53-year-old woman undergoing hepatico-jejunostomy. **a** MIP-reconstructed MRCP image shows a tight stenosis of the anastomosis with moderate dilation of the intrahepatic ducts. **b** Source image allows the correct evaluation of the site of the anastomosis, showing the relationship between the hepatic ducts and the intestinal loop. Also, the size and the extension of the stenosis is better visualized

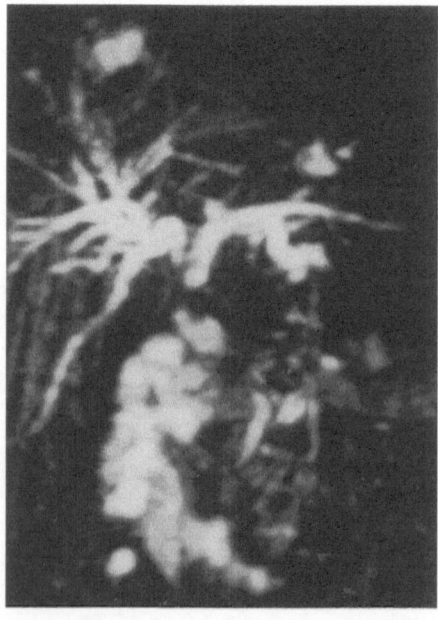

a

**Fig. 5** (cont.)

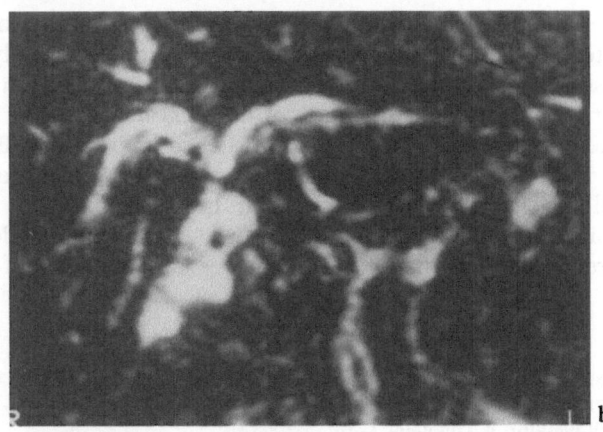

**Fig. 6 a,b.** 52-year-old woman treated with hepatico-jejunostomy. **a** MIP-reconstructed MRCP image shows a filling defect at the level of the anastomosis, with wide dilation of the intrahepatic ducts. **b** Source image depicts the presence of 1.8-cm stone wedged at the level of the anastomosis and multiple stones in the intrahepatic ducts

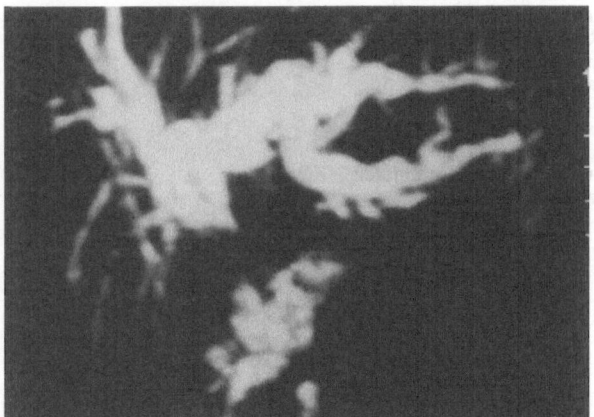

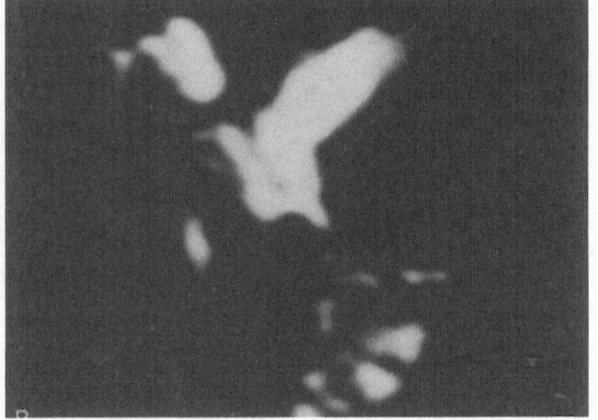

In comparison with biliscintigraphy, some limitations of MRCP may be related to the lack of functional information, especially in differentiating persistent postsurgical bile duct dilation from dilation related to current obstruction. In addition, signs of mild cholangitis may be misdiagnosed due to the poor spatial resolution of MRCP compared with ERCP and PTC.

In conclusion, MRCP is a safe, noninvasive technique for the evaluation of biliary-enteric anastomosis with high accuracy in assessing the cause of jaundice. MRCP images may be used as a guide following an interventional procedure. The main disadvantages are the lack of functional information

**Fig. 7 a–d.** A 49-year-old woman undergoing hepatico-jejunostomy. **a** The axial T2-weighted turbo spin echo image shows dilation of the intrahepatic ducts with multiple intraluminal hypointense images suggesting stones. **b** MIP-reconstructed MRCP image offers a panoramic evaluation of the dilated ducts with a "filling defect" at the level of the anastomosis. **c,d** Source images demonstrate multiple stones, ranging in diameter between 1 and 2 cm

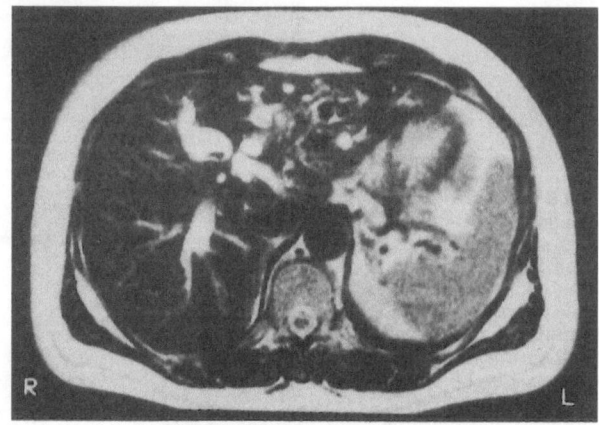

a

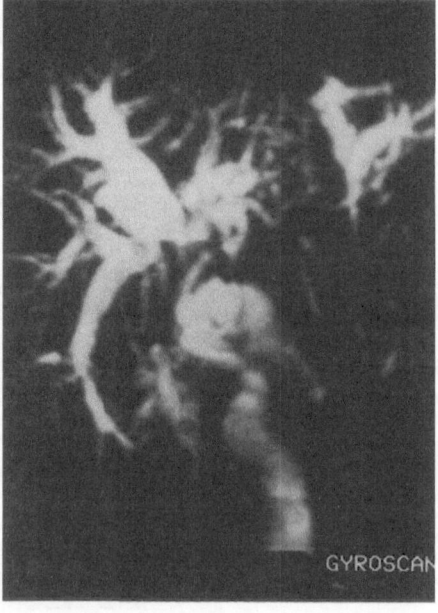

b

**Fig. 7** (cont.)

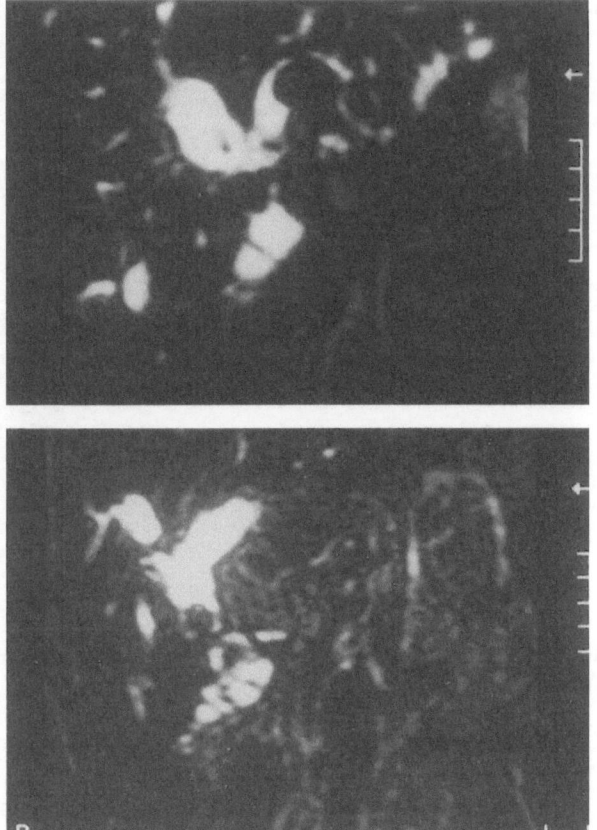

c

d

**Fig. 8 a,b.** A 52-year-old man undergoing hepatico-jejunostomy. **a** MIP-reconstructed image shows dilation of the intrahepatic ducts, in particular on the left segments. **b** the evaluation of the source images demonstrates multpile small stones in the hepatic ducts

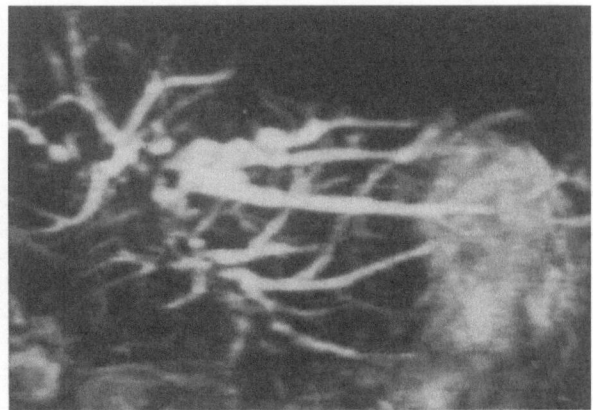

a

**Fig. 8** (cont.)

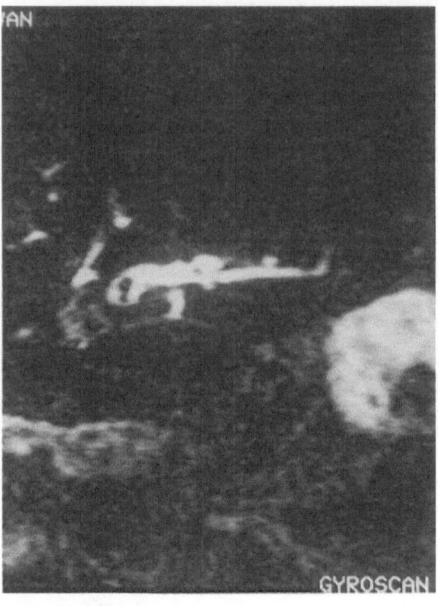

b

and the high cost, which limits its use as a screening study in symptomatic patients.

## Personal Experience

At our institution we have studied 15 patients (8 men and 7 women) aged 49–80 years (mean 64.7). The types of anastomotic procedures include hepatico-jejunostomy ($n$=13) and choledocho-duodenostomy ($n$=2). Indications for imaging studies included scheduled follow-up ($n$=7), persistent jaundice ($n$=4), cholangitis and abnormal liver function tests ($n$=2), and combination

**Fig. 9 a,b.** A 64-year-old woman treated with choledocho-duodenostomy. **a** MIP-reconstructed MRCP image shows dilation of the CBD and the intrahepatic ducts, with no evidence of filling defect inside the CBD. Native choledochus is well represented. **b** Single slice evaluation shows the presence of a 0.5-cm stone at the level of the proximal third of CBD

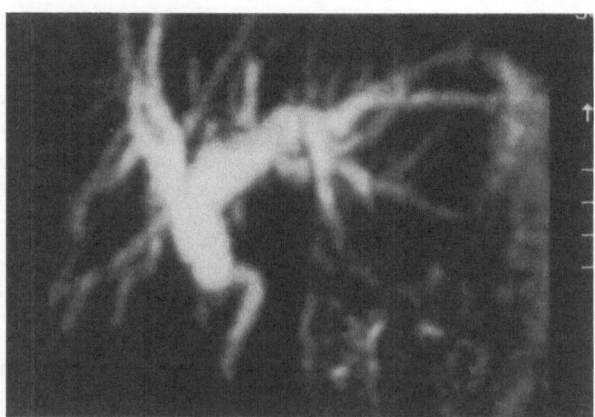

a

**Fig. 9** (cont.)

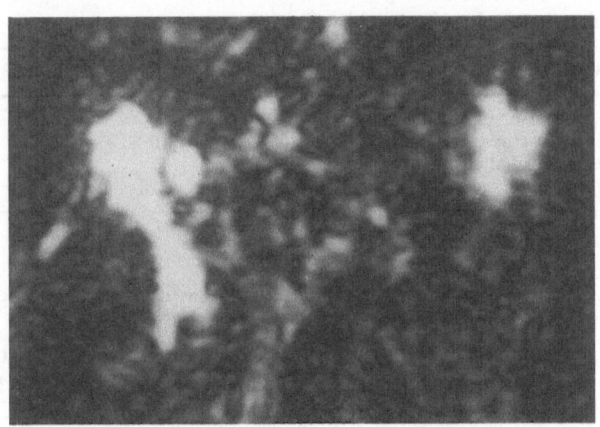

b

of transient jaundice, epigastric pain, abnormal liver function tests in the remaining two.

Six patients were subsequently evaluated by means of PTC to confirm the diagnosis and to perform a therapeutic procedure. Two patients undergoing choledocho-duodenostomy were evaluated by ERCP. The remaining eight patients studied as part of their surgical follow-up and presenting no significant symptoms or dilation of the bile ducts were not treated by any invasive procedure.

Image quality was graded as good in nine cases (60%), fair in three (20%), and poor in the remaining three (20%). $k$ values for measurement of interobserver agreement were excellent for the evaluation of dilated bile ducts ($k=1$), stenosis of the anastomosis ($k=0.86$), and stones ($k=0.92$) and good for the assessment of signs of cholangitis ($k=0.59$; Tables 1, 2).

The value of MRCP in these patients is confirmed by the following data:
- Dilation of bile ducts: In all the eight patients presenting with either severe or mild dilation of intrahepatic ducts MRCP provided a correct assessment of the degree of dilation, with a complete agreement between the observers. In the remaining seven patients with no dilated ducts MRCP provided a correct visualization of the anastomosis and the main hepatic ducts.
- Signs of cholangitis: In the eight patients affected by cholangitis MRCP correcly showed bile ducts irregularities in two. There were two false-nega-

**Table 1.** Interobserver agreement

| Type of lesion | Total lesions | Observed agreement | Agreement expected by chance | Overall $k$ value |
|---|---|---|---|---|
| Evidence of bile ducts | 15 | 1 | 0.37 | 1 |
| Signs of cholangitis | 8 | 0.87 | 0.68 | 0.59 |
| Stenosis of the anastomosis | 15 | 0.93 | 0.50 | 0.86 |
| Stones | 5 | 0.93 | 0.14 | 0.92 |

**Table 2.** Results obtained by first observer

| Type of lesions | TP | TN | FP | FN | Total |
|---|---|---|---|---|---|
| Evidence of bile ducts | 8 | 7 | 0 | 0 | 15 |
| Signs of cholagitis | 6 | 7 | 0 | 2 | 15 |
| Stenosis of the anastomosis | 8 | 7 | 0 | 0 | 15 |
| Stones | 5 | 10 | 0 | 0 | 15 |

tive results due to poor spatial resolution of the technique. Agreement was not as good as that in cases of dilation ($k=0.59$).
- Stenosis of the anastomosis: In eight patients there was stenosis of the anastomosis, and this was correctly evaluated by MRCP in each case, with an excellent agreement ($k=0.86$).
- Stones: 5–15 mm stones were identified in five patients. Stones were wedged at the level of the anastomoses ($n=2$) or were localized in the intrahepatic ducts ($n=4$). Multiple stones were observed in four of the five patients. Only a 5-mm stone, in a patient with choledocho-duodenostomy, was missed by one observer, but it was correctly evaluated by the other ($k=0.92$).

## References

1.  Halleb A, Frileux P, Cohen JP et al (1986) Fistules bilio-biliaires d'origine lithiasique. A propos de huit cas. Ann Chir 40:363–366
2.  Bismuth H, Lazorthes F (1981) Les traumatismes operatoires de la voie biliare principale. Masson, Paris
3.  Bismuth H (1982) Postoperative stricture of the bile duct. In: Blumgarth LM (ed) The biliary tract. Churchill Livingstone, Edinburgh, pp 209–218
4.  Blumgart LH, Kelley CJ, Benjamin IS (1984) Benign bile duct stricture following cholecystectomy: critical factors in management. Br J Surg 71:836–843
5.  Machado MCC, Monteiro Da Cunha JE, Bacchella T (1986) A modified technique for surgical repair of cicatricial stenosis of the bile duct. Surg Gynec Obstet 162:283–284
6.  Pitt HA, Miyamoto T, Parapatis SK et al (1982) Factors influencing outcome in patients with postoperative biliary strictures. Am J Surg 144:14–18
7.  Voiles CR, Blumgart LH (1982) A technique for the construction of high biliary-enteric anastomoses. Surg Gynecol Obstet 154:885–887
8.  Huguier M, Houry S, Lacaine F, Pascal G (1986) Les anastomoses choledoco-duodenales dans la lithiasesa biliaire. J Chir 123:3–6
9.  Bismuth H, Franco D, Corlette MB, Hepp J (1978) Long term results of Roux-en-Y hepaticojejunostomy. Surg Gynecol Obstet 146:161–167
10. Hepp J, Bismuth H (1966) Accidents et complications precoces de la sphincterotomie odienne. Rev Int Hepatol 16:497–519
11. Lane CE, Sawyers JL, Riddell DH (1973) Long-term results of Roux-en-Y hepatocholangiojejunostomy. Ann Surg 177:714–720
12. Stefanini P, Carboni M, Patrassi N et al (1975) Roux-en-y hepaticojejunostomy: a reappraisal of its indications and results. Ann Surg 181:213–219
13. Genest JF, Nanos E, Grundfest-Broniatowsky S et al (1986) Benign biliary strictures: an analytic review (1979–1984). Surgery 99:409–413
14. Eubanks B, Martinex CR, Mehigan D, Cameron GL (1982) Current role of intravenous cholangiography. Am J Surg 143:731–733
15. Negrin JA, Zanzi I, Margouleff D (1995) Hepatobiliary scintigraphy after biliary tract surgery. Semin Nucl Med 25:28–35
16. Wilson SR, Toi A (1990) Sonography accurately detects biliary obstruction in patients with surgically created biliary-enteric anastomosis. AJR 155:789–794

17. Montalvo BM, Fanney DR, Yrizarry JM, Russell E (1989) Hepaticodochojejunostomy with afferent limb: CT anatomy. Gastrointest Radiol 14:246–250
18. Tidmore H, Ram MD (1985) Scintiscanning in the evaluation of biliary-enteric anastomoses. Ann Surg 51:158–161
19. Palmer Gold R, Price JB (1980) The thin needle cholangiography as the primary method for the evaluation of the biliary-enteric anastomosis. Radiology 136:309–316
20. Papp J, Tulassay Z, Bielawski J et al (1977) Diagnostic value of endoscopic retrograde cholangiopancreatography in bilio-digestive anastomoses. Acta Hepatogastroenterol 24:41–43
21. Hamilton I, Lintott DJ, Rothwell J, Axon ATR (1983) Acute pancreatitis following endoscopic retrograde cholangiopancreatography. Clin Radiol 34:543–546
22. Morimoto K, Shimoi M, Shirakawa T et al (1992) Biliary obstruction: evaluation with three-dimensional MR cholangiography. Radiology 183:578–580
23. Guibaud L, Bret PM, Reinhold C et al (1995) Bile duct obstruction and choledocholithiasis: diagnosis with MR cholangiography. Radiology 197:109–115
24. Pavone P, Laghi A, Catalano C et al (1995) Three-dimensional MR cholangiography: a unique diagnostic procedure for evaluation of bile ducts in patients with biliary-enteric anastomoses. Radiology 197:312

# CHAPTER 10

# MRCP in Liver-Transplanted Patients

## Introduction

Biliary complications remain an important problem following liver transplantation [1, 2]. The frequency of biliary complications ranges between 15% and 20% of cases, although a recent study has reported a rate of 11.5% [3-7]. The complication rate depends also on the type of anastomotic procedure, for example, bilio-biliary termino-terminal anastomosis or bilio-digestive choledocho-jejunal anastomosis, the former being preferred due to the decreased risk of infection (cholangitis) and the conservation of the sphincter of Oddi [8].

Most complications occur within the first month, although late complications can be observed years after transplantation [1, 9]. The former are bile leakage while the latter are mainly stenoses of the CBD at the level of the anastomosis. A particular type of complication is the so-called "ampullary dysfunction," where an isolated dilatation of the extrahepatic ducts occurs, probably related to denervation of the papilla during the hepatectomy. This kind of complication occurs in up to 16.6% of patients.

## Etiology and Location of Biliary Strictures in Transplanted Patients

Recently the etiology of various involvements of the biliary tree in transplanted patients has received particular attention. There is a difference between the strictures appearing at the level of the anastomosis and the intrahepatic strictures. Anastomotic strictures are encountered more frequently (up to 15% of cases), and their etiology has been classically related to a simple excessive fibrotic reaction at the anastomosis. However, various causes must be considered due to the higher incidence of strictures in these patients than in those undergoing biliary anastomosis without transplantation. The evidence that ischemia at the donor site must be considered comes from evaluation of the incidence of intrahepatic strictures. Intrahepatic strictures have recently been reported to occur with an incidence of 8.2% [10]. The cause of the intrahepatic strictures have been directly correlated to ischemia of the donor's liver. There is a higher incidence in patients with hepatic artery occlusion. Another cause is the so-called "cold ischemia" that occurs during the period between cross-clamping of liver vessels in the donor and allograft reperfusion in the recipient [11]. Bile duct epithelial injury occurs during prolonged cold ischemia [12].

An alternative etiology is the presence of a chronic hepatic damage (chronic rejection) [13, 14]. Chronic rejection causes ischemic changes of chronic obliterative arteriopathy, and the resulting ischemia may lead to bile duct epithelial injury.

Treatment of the stricures is based on the degree of bile obstruction. In intrahepatic strictures retransplantation must also be considered, as an alternative to percutaneous dilatation. Campbell [15] describes a 3% rate of retransplantation and a 56% rate of percutaneous treatment.

## Determining the Presence of Biliary Stricture

Noninvasive methods must be employed in evaluating these patients. The symptoms are not always specific, and a suspected stenosis is often not found at cholangiographic evaluation. Therefore we must try to limit the use of ERCP, which is currently the technique of choice for evaluation of these patients.

Ultrasound has limited sensitivity, although it remains a first-line examination, especially in detecting fluid collections secondary to bile leakage. Less accurate is the evaluation of the stenotic anastomosis or the dilation of the CBD until the level of the papilla. CT may be useful in the case of fistula to assess fluid collections, but CT assesment of the bile ducts does not provide a correct evaluation of the stenosis of the anastomosis. Thus a direct cholangiographic view of the bile ducts is mandatory to obtain a correct diagnosis and to plan an adequate treatment. Opacification of the bile ducts has a sensitivity of 100% and provides a correct assessment of the lesions. Transhepatic cholangiography is preferable to retrograde opacification due to the risks of infection, although each technique has a known morbidity and mortality.

Biliary strictures that develop in the early phases after transplantation may be evaluated by direct cholangiographic study through a T-tube. However, more often the complication occurs in a later stage, when no T-tube is present, and a different approach must be considered. In defining intrahepatic stenosis Campbell uses percutaneus biliary puncture and evaluation in more than 60% of cases. Limiting the use of this approach in this group of patients is the goal of MRCP.

## Role of MRCP

We have evaluated the possible role of MRCP in the follow-up of liver transplanted patients. The use of MRCP is of course limited to late complications because bile leakage after ultrasound or CT demonstration of the fluid collection requires a percutaneous or endoscopic approach to perform a therapeutic intervention (biliary drainage; drainage of the fluid collection).

**Fig. 1.** MRCP showing CBD stenosis at the level of the anastomosis

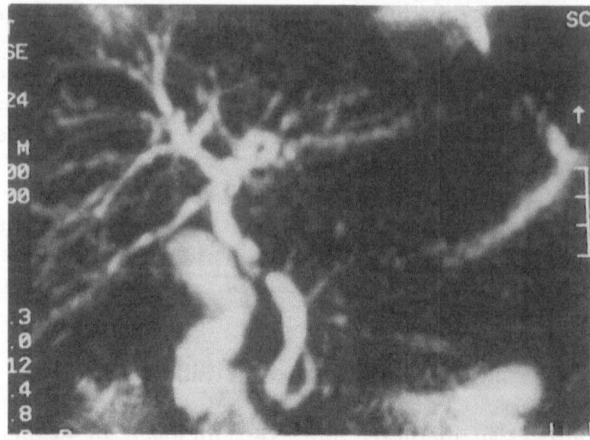

**Fig. 2. a** Axial T2-weighted MR image showing dilation of the left intrahepatic branches. **b** MRCP shows stenosis involving only the left hepatic duct

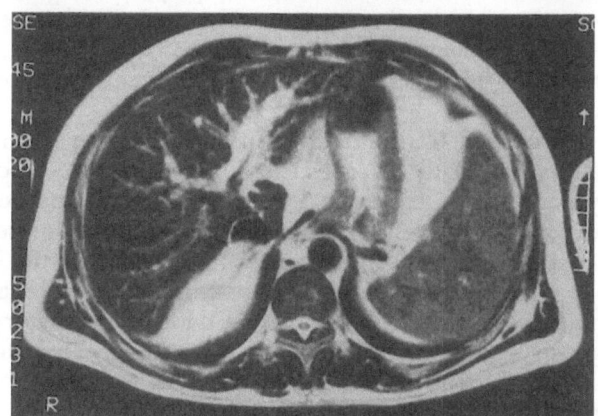

a

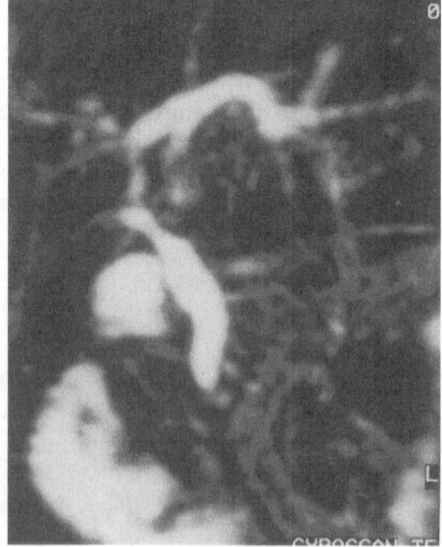

b

**Fig. 3.** Tight stenosis at the level of the confluence of the hepatic ducts, with wide dilation of the intrahepatic branches

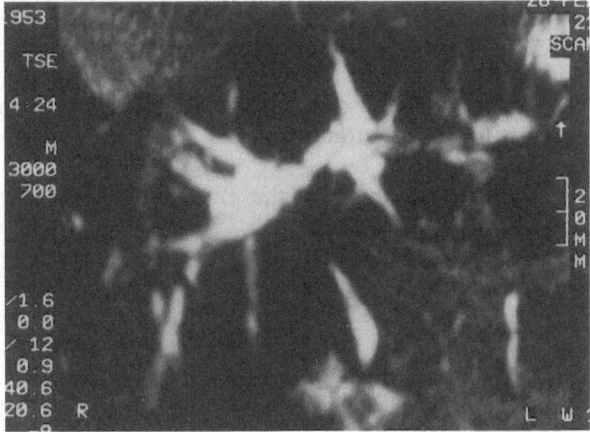

In late complications (e.g., stenosis or ampullary dysfunction) MRCP may have an important role due to the lack of invasivity of this technique. Patients with alterations in liver function results may be studied by MRCP in to obtain direct representation of the biliary tract, with a correct assessment of the patency of the anastomosis, the presence of a possible stenosis, and the dilation of the intrahepatic bile ducts. Furthermore, a diagnosis of ampullary dysfunction can be proposed without any invasivity due to the complete representation of the extrahepatic ducts possible in all the cases.

The definition of the site and extent of the stenosis can be obtained directly by MRCP (Fig. 1). The lack of signal in the area of the stenosis may lead to an overestimation of the stenosis itself. However, this is not a crucial

**Fig. 4.** MRCP performed after PTC-guided drainage; a slight dilation of the intrahepatic ducts is still evident

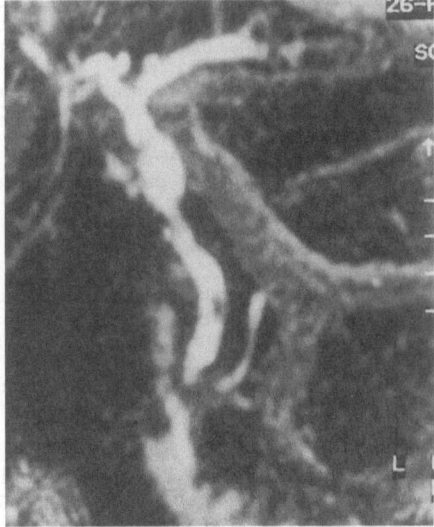

point. The decision of whether to perform any treatment is taken mostly on the basis of the clinical symptoms and on the alteration of liver enzymes, in addition to the morphology of the duct above the anastomotic level. In extensive dilatation the decision is to treat, while in mild dilatation and limited changes in the functional tests no treatment is given, but follow-up is undertaken (Fig. 2).

In addition to showing the evidence of the morphology of the bile ducts at the anastomosis, MRCP may provide a complete map of the intrahepatic ducts (Figs. 3, 4). The evidence of intrahepatic bile ducts strictures is a relevant issue and requires treatment in most of the patients, even in the absence of anastomotic dilatation. Using a noninvasive modality such as MRCP allows screening for patients with symptoms but not affected by significant stricures. In our experience this occurs in more than 30% of cases. In some patients it is possible to evaluate the presence of other causes of biliary dysfunction, such as a papillitis, since the "ampullary dysfuntion" is evident in 16.6% of cases and related to peroperative ischemia. With a clear map of the anatomy of the bile ducts the surgeon is able to evaluate the extent of the biliary involvement and to select the appropriate treatment, if any.

## References

1. Iwatsuki S, Shaw BW Jr, Starlz TE (1983) Biliary tract comlpications in liver transplantation under cyclosporin-steroid therapy. Transplant Proc 15:1288–1291
2. Starzl TE, Putnam CW, Hansbrough JF et al (1977) Biliary complications after liver transplantation: with special reference to the biliary cast syndrome and techniques of secondary duct repair. Surgery 81:212–21
3. D'Alessandro AM, Kalajoglu M, Pirsch JD et al (1991) Biliary tract complications after orthotopic liver transplantation. Transplant Proc 23:1956
4. Lebeau G, Yanaga K, Marsh JW et al (1990) Analysis of surgical complications after 397 hepatic transplantation. Surg Gynecol Obstet 170:317–22
5. Ringe B. Oldhafer K, Buzendah H et al (1989) Analysis of biliary complications following orthotopic liver transplantation. Transplant Proc 21:2472–76
6. Stratta RJ, Wood RP, Langas AN et al (1989) Diagnosis and treatment of biliary tract complications after orthotopic liver transplantation. Surgery 106:675–84
7. Turrion VS, Mora NP, Herrera J et al (1992) Surgical aspects of the first 150 liver transplants as a multicenter program in Madrid. Transplant Proc 24:158–159
8. Krom RAF, Kingma LM, Wesenhagen H et al (1984) Choledochocholedochostomy is successful in orthotopic liver transplantation. Transplant Proc 16:1228–1229
9. Greif F, Bronsther OL, Van Thieil DH et al (1994) The incidence, timing and management of biliary tract complications after orthotpic liver transplantation. Ann Surg 219:40–45
10. Campbell WL, Sheng R, Zajko AB et. al (1994) Intrahepatic biliary strictures after liver transplantation. Radiology 191:735–740
11. Sanchez Urdazpal L, Gores GJ, Ward EM et al (1992) Ischemic-type biliary complications after orthotopic liver transplantation Hepatology 16:49–53
12. McMaster P, Herbertson B, Cusick C, Calne RY, Williams R (1978) Biliary sludging following liver transplantation in man. Transplantation 25:56–62
13. Ward EM, Kiely MJ, Masus TP, Wiesner RH, Krom RAF (1990) Hilar biliary strictures after liver transplantation: cholangiography and percutaneous treatment. Radiology 177:259–263
14. McDonald V, Matalon TAS, Patel SK et al (1991) Biliary strictures in hepatic transplantation.
15. Miller WJ, Campbell WL, Zajko AB et al (1991) Obstructive dilatation of extrahepatic recipient and donor bile ducts complicating orthotopic liver transplantation: imaging and laboratory findings. AJR 157:29–32

# CHAPTER 11

# The Role of ERCP in the Era of MRCP

## Introduction

MRCP will in the future modify the approach to patients affected with biliary or pancreatic pathologies. Preliminary results show high sensitivity in detecting benign or malignant lesions affecting the biliary tree and related organs. Considering the predominant role of ERCP in this pathology, both diagnostic and therapeutic, it is likely to that there will be changes in ERCP indications – restricting the diagnostic ones but totally maintaining the therapeutic. This brief chapter considers the residual role of ERCP, presuming a future widespread use of MRCP.

## MRCP: Advantages and Disadvantages

MRCP presents some clear advantages over ERCP. First of all, it is a totally noninvasive technique and is therefore well tolerated by patients and is repeatable. This enables it to be used even in patients presenting with poor symptoms.

MRCP is less expensive than ERCP, including the factors of endoscopist, radiology unit, and technicians. In the United States the costs of ERCP are estimated at twice those of MRCP. In Italy, as in Europe generally, there is a lack of MR equipment in public health, which is overloaded by neuroradiology or osteoarticular routine. This trend will be probably modified by MRCP and other abdominal MR implications.

A further advantage of MRCP is to extend diagnostic information from the simple biliopancreatic duct morphology to the surroundings structures, such as parenchymal, vascular, and adipose tissues. MRCP thus has the advantage to condense into a unique technique the diagnostic power of the direct visualization of the biliary tree, as with ERCP, and the study of the parenchyma, providing similar or better results than CT.

Among the limitations of MRCP is its inferior spatial resolution which does not allow identification of the thinest morphological alterations (e.g., pancreatic branches). In addition, MRCP yields poor-quality images in the absence of biliary tree dilatation. Lastly, MRCP does not enable functional studies; however, this kind of evaluation is easily obtained by biliary scintigraphy.

## ERCP: Advantages and Disadvantages

As noted above, some of the ERCP characteristics ensure it a residual role in the diagnostic evaluation of biliary and pancreatic ducts lesions. First of all, ERCP has the undeniable advantage of providing a detailed map of the biliary tree with a better spatial resolution than MRCP. This advantage is less remarkable in the study of CBD, Wirsung duct, or Vater ampulla, but it is quite important with the intrahepatic ducts, especially if they are not dilated, and the thinnest intraparenchymal pancreatic branches.

ERCP can visualize biliopancreatic ducts even in the absence of dilatation, and it provides important functional information (e.g., contrast medium emptying at the end of the diagnostic phase) [1, 2]. This advantage can in any case be considered of lesser importance as in almost all biliary pathologies these is a certain degree of dilatation that can be easily detected by ultrasound. Theoricaly, on the basis of ultrasound results in relation to biliary dilatation, ERCP or MRCP is indicated.

A further advantage of ERCP is the chance to proceed immediately to therapeutic procedures, performing an endoscopic sphincterotomy or biliary stenting [3, 4]. While this seems a clear advantage, the therapeutic approach offered by ERCP is not always the best for the patient, as in case of occasionally unsatisfactory clinical results following the frequent endoscopic sphincterotomy and in cases of stenting of neoplastic lesions that may later be resected.

In addition, as for percutaneous cholangiography, there is great difficulty in evaluating the remnant biliary tree in case of strict stenoses. We therefore obtain only a partial study of the biliary tree. MRCP, on the other hand, always enables a complete evaluation.

## Residual Role of ERCP

In conclusion, we can consider a residual role for diagnostic ERCP in the following cases:
- In the absence of biliary tree dilatation, if symptoms require a complete evaluation of the biliary tree
- To evaluate the thinnest anatomic changes, such as in the study of intrahepatic ducts or pancreatic branches
- If ultrasound shows CBD stones, as in this case the indication is already therapeutic.

## References

1.   Varley PF, Rohrmann CA Jr, Silvis SE, Vennes JA (1976) The normal endoscopic pancreatogram. Radiology 118:295–300
2.   Schapiro RH (1989) ERCP in the diagnosis of pancreatic and biliary disease. In: Schapiro RH (ed) ERCP: diagnostic and therapeutic applications. Elsevier, New York, pp 9–40
3.   Siegel JH (1991) Endoscopic retrograde cholangio-pancreatography: technique, diagnosis, and therapy. Raven, New York, pp 52–56
4.   Cotton PB, Williams CB (1990) ERCP. In practical gastrointestinal endoscopy. Blackwell, Oxford, pp 85–117

# MRCP in the Evaluation of Choledocholithiasis Prior to Laparoscopic Cholecystectomy

## Introduction

Since 1987, when Mouret performed the first laparoscopic cholecystectomy, there has been a remarkable change in the surgical treatment of gallstones [1]. In most centers laparoscopic cholecystectomy has become the procedure of choice for symptomatic cholelithiasis [2]. The laparoscopic approach is more acceptable due to lower morbidity, reduced postoperative pain, lower cost, shorter hospital stay, and earlier return to work. Because of the limited contraindications (e.g., severe acute peritonitis, severe portal hypertension, carcinoma of the gallbladder, coagulopathies, third trimester of pregnancy) about 95% of patients with gallstones are treated by laparoscopic cholecystectomy [3].

The new therapeutic approach has brought new diagnostic needs related to the evaluation of the associated choledocholithiasis, which has been demonstrated in 3%–33% of patients, according to various authors [4]. Several studies have examined the problem related to choledocholithiasis, but there is no consensus regarding diagnosis or therapy. From the therapeutic point of view, preoperative diagnosis of CBD stones requires either a conversion to an open operation or attempted laparoscopic extraction or leaving the calculi in situ with either a subsequent endoscopic sphincterotomy or conservative management [5]. Currently most authors prefer a preoperative endoscopic procedure, with a laparoscopic exploration of the CBD restricted to selected patients [6].

## Preoperative Evaluation

At the preoperative stage various techniques have been proposed for the evaluation of choledocholithiasis: abdominal ultrasound, CT, intravenous cholangiography, and ERCP. A different approach to evaluating the possible presence of stones is to perform an intraoperative study by cholangiography and/or ultrasound. Abdominal ultrasound has an overall sensitivity of 55% in detecting CBD stones, but if the diameter of the CBD is less than 6 mm (in up to 86% of patients) stones cannot be detected. CT has been widely evaluated in the past as a noninvasive screening method in diagnosing CBD stones, with sensitivity reported between 83% and 90% [8, 9], but more recent studies [10] have found lower sensitivity (75%). The major limitation of preoperative intravenous cholangiography is the lack of opacification of the biliary system (30%–40% of cases). In a prospective study intravenous cholangiography was useful in detecting choledocholithiasis in only 1.5% of cases [11]. Moreover, there are risks related to adverse reaction of contrast agents, high costs, and poor anatomic definition of the intra- and extrahepatic bile ducts [12].

The use of ERCP prior to a laparoscopic cholecystectomy is controversial. Good results have been obtained by combining ERCP and endoscopic sphincterotomy in the diagnosis and management of suspected CBD stones. However, patient selection is very important because 10% of patients who undergo this procedure develop some type of complication, with a mortality of 0.37%–1.0% [13]. Even if ERCP cannot be considered as a screening procedure in preoperative evaluation of patients with suspected CBD stones, it can be performed if a high clinical suspicion for the presence of stones is evident.

Several authors use a series of clinical, laboratory, and radiological indicators to determine the presence of stones [14, 15]. A direct correlation between the number of positive criteria and the presence of stones has been established. However, in the better series 4%–10% of patients with CBD stones are not detected due to the lack of symptoms.

## Intraoperative Evaluation

The second approach is to perform an intraoperative study by intraoperative cholangiography and ultrasonography. Intraoperative cholangiography performed during a laparoscopic procedure is inconvenient, time-consuming, and potentially harmful because a bile duct injury can occur [16]. Intraoperative cholangiography therefore does not appear to have a role unless the demonstration of stones in the duct leads to immediate exploration of the CBD, which is a technically difficult procedure. Laparoscopic ultrasonography has some limitations due to technical problems and can be considered as an ancillary technique to intraoperative cholangiography.

## MRCP for Detecting CBD Stones Before Laparoscopic Cholecystectomy

Recent studies have reported a high reliability of MRCP in detecting stones in the CBD. A larger series showed a sensitivity of 88% and a specificity of 98%, a positive predictive value of 91%, a negative predictive value of 97%, and an overall diagnostic accuracy of 96%.

We conducted a study among 40 patients undergoing laparoscopic chlecystectomy (14 men, 26 women; age 28–72 years, mean 54). The patients were studied with MRCP to evaluate the presence of CBD stones. Inclusion criteria, other than the known gallbladder stones, were one or more of the following: previous episodes of jaundice, increased alkaline phosphatase, and dilation of bile ducts at ultrasound. MRCP was performed 2–4 days prior to surgery. In all patients intraoperative cholangiography was performed during the laparoscopic procedure for diagnostic confirmation and for a therapeutic

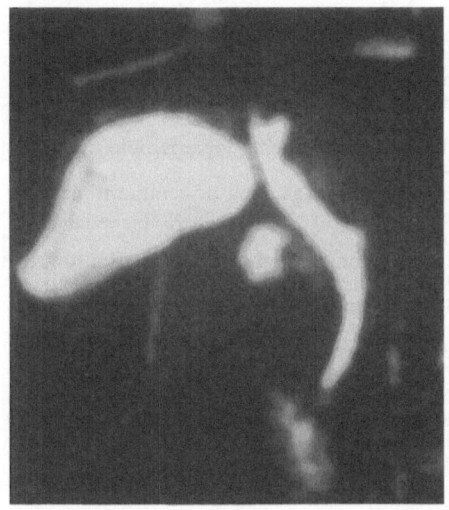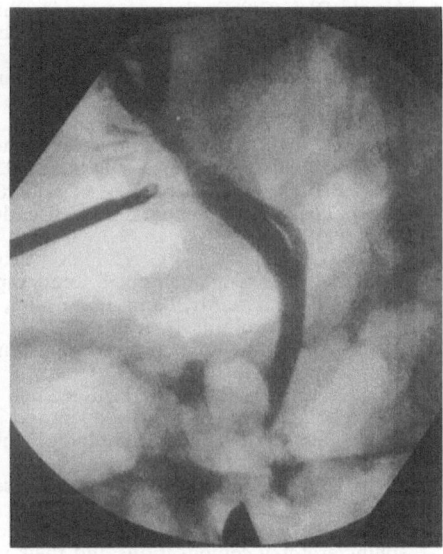

a                                                                              b

**Fig. 1a,b.** Patient with known gallbladder stones. **a** On MRCP on MIP-reconstructed image an inhomogeneous signal is appreciable at the distal tract of the CBD. **b** On the source image the stone is clearly evident

approach, when necessary. Of the 40 patients 23 (57.5%) had CBD stones, as confirmed at intraoperative procedure. MRCP correctly evaluated all of these 23 cases (Fig. 1).

## Role of MRCP

Despite its high accuracy in detecting CBD stones MRCP cannot be considered as a screening technique to be performed in all patients prior to surgery due to the high costs of the procedure. It should be confined to patients with positive predictive factors. The accuracy of the predictive factors is less good. Enzymes values each have an accuracy of 17%–22%; jaundice is present in a minority of patients, and ultrasound is able to detect CBD stones in only 23%–80%. In a large surgical series of 950 patients, 100 presented stones at intraoperative cholangiography, but the predictive signs were positive in only 66%.

## References

1. Mouret (1991) From the first laparoscopic cholecystectomy to the frontiers of laparoscopic surgery: the future prospectives. Dig Surg 8:124–125
2. Franceschi D, Brandt C, Margolin D, Szopa B, Ponsky J, Priebe P, Stellato T, Eckhauser ML (1993) The management of common bile duct stones in patients undergoing laparoscopic cholecystectomy. Am Surg 59:525–532
3. National Institute of Health Consensus Development Conference Statement on Gallstones and Laparoscopic Cholecystectomy (1993). Am J Surg 165:390–398

4. Arnold DJ (1970) Cholecystectomy in Ohio: results of a survey in Ohio hospital by the Gallbladder Survey Committee, Ohio Chapter, American College of Surgeons. Am J Surg 119:714–717
5. Patel JC, McInnes GC, Bagley JS, Needham G, Krukowski ZH (1993) The role of intravenous cholangiography in pre-operative assessment for laparoscopic cholecystectomy. Br J Radiol 66:1125–1127
6. Berci G (1991) Cholangiography and choledochoscopy during laparoscopic cholecystectomy, its place and value. Dig Surg 8:92–96
7. Gross BH, Harter LP, Gore RM et al (1983) Ultrsonic evaluation of common bile duct stones. Prospective comparison with endoscopic retrograde cholangiopancreatography. Radiology 146:471
8. Baron RL, Stanley RJ, Lee JKT (1982) Prospective comparison of the evaluation of biliary obstruction using computed tomography and ultrasonography. Radiology 145:91
9. Jeffrey RB, Federle MP, Laing FC, Wall S, Rego J, Moss AA (1983) Computed tomography in choledocolithiasis. AJR 140:1179
10. Baron RL (1987) Common bile ducts stones. Reassessment of criteria for CT diagnosis. Radiology 162:419
11. Patel, McInnes G C, Bagley JS, Needham G, Krukowski ZH (1993) The role of intravenous cholangiography in pre-operative assessment for laparoscopic cholecystectomy. Departments of Diagnostic Radiology and Surgery, Aberdeeen Royal Infirmary, Foresterhill, Aberdeen
12. Shehadi WH, Toniolo G (1980) Adverse reaction to contrast media. Diagn Radiol 137:299–302
13. Cotton PB, Lehman G, Vennes J, Geenen JE, Russell RCG et al (1991) Endoscopic sphincterotomy complications and their management: an attempt at consensus. Gastrointest Endosc 37:383–393
14. Reis R, Deutsch AA, Nudelman I, Kott I (1984) Statistical value of various clinical parameters in predicting the presence of choledochal stones. Surg Gynecol Obstet 159:273–276
15. Hauer-Jensen M, Karesen R, Nygaard K, Solheim K, Amlie E et al (1985) Predictive ability of choledocholithiasis indicators: a prospective evaluation. Ann Surg 202:64–68
16. Grogono JL, Woods WGA (1986) Selective use of operative cholangiography. World J Surg 10:1009–1013

# MR Cholangiography in the Postoperative Evaluation of Patients Undergoing Laparoscopic Cholecystectomy

## Introduction

Gallbladder stones is one of the most widespread diseases worldwide. In the United States alone 500 000 cholecystectomies are performed every year [1]. Laparoscopic cholecystectomy is the current accepted surgical procedure for the treatment of gallbladder stones; this innovative technique was first proposed in 1987 by Mouret. The laparoscopic procedures performed for cholecystectomy are relatively standardized, and all surgical centers in the world have accepted them [2–4].

In addition to perioperative complications, recurrent symptoms may arise after laparoscopic cholecystectomy and may be due to a number of causes, including residual stones in the main bile duct and iatrogenic lesions of the bile ducts. These are the most feared complications, and their incidence varies with the experience of the surgeon. Values ranging between 0.6 and 0.16 are reported in literature [5–8].

Diagnostic evaluation in symptomatic patients following laparoscopic cholecystectomy requires a complete overview of the status of the biliary tree. ERCP is usually performed for this. However, symptoms are often mild (recurrent colic), no treatment is generally required, and the use of a relatively invasive procedure as ERCP is not welcomed either by the patient or the surgeon.

MR cholangiography can also play a diagnostic role in patients undergoing previous laparoscopic cholecystectomy; titanium clips present no problems. We evaluated the MRCP findings in a series of patients with symptoms after laparoscopic cholecystectomy, in which MRCP was performed as primary diagnostic modality.

## Personal Series

We used MRCP to examine 34 patients (mean age 56 years) with recurrent symptoms after laparoscopic cholecystectomy. Surgery had been performed between 10 days and 2 years previously by various groups of surgeons (our hospital is a referring center for biliary disease). Symptoms included dyspepsia, nausea and vomiting, pain and recurrent colic, and recurrent episodes of jaundice.

ERCP was performed in 14 patients following MRCP and transhepatic biliary drainage in 8. In 17 cases an interventional procedure was performed (9 by endoscopic approach and 8 by percutaneous transhepatic approach). In 10 cases the biliary tree was evaluated only with MRCP. These cases, presenting with mild symptoms, were followed up clinically and no further diagnostic or interventional procedure was performed. In these cases the biliary tree was normal.

Recurrent bile duct stones were found in six patients, three of which also presented a significant dilatation of the bile ducts. The stones ranged in diameter between 3 and 8 mm and were located in the distal bile duct in five and at the hepatic ducts confluence in one. Stones were evident in the MIP-reconstructed images in four cases, while only the evaluation of the single slices allowed detection of the stones in the remaining cases. In all these patients ERCP was performed following MRCP and removal of stones was per-

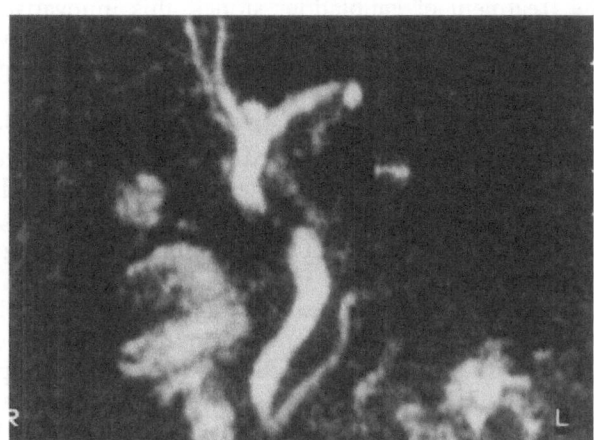

**Fig. 1.** MRCP image shows iatrogenic stricture of the CBD located more than 2 cm from the carrefour

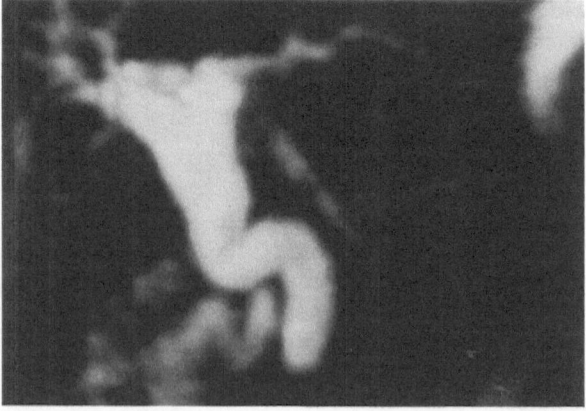

**Fig. 2.** MRCP image shows a wide dilation of the CBD with a distal smooth narrowing at ampulla

**Fig. 3.** MRCP of papillitis
with moderately dilated biliary tract that shrinks distally to the flute beak

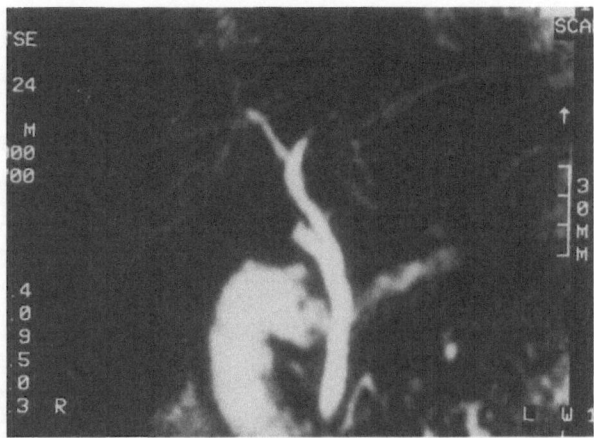

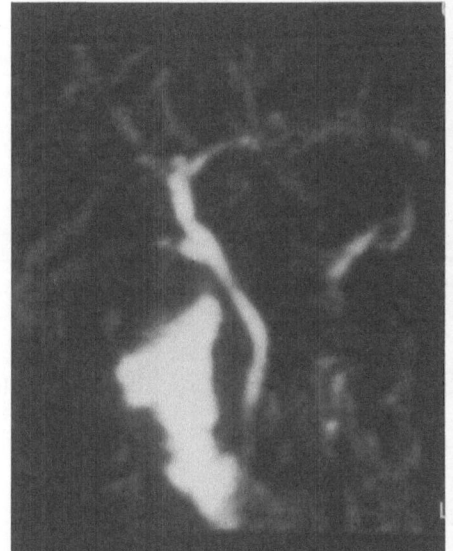
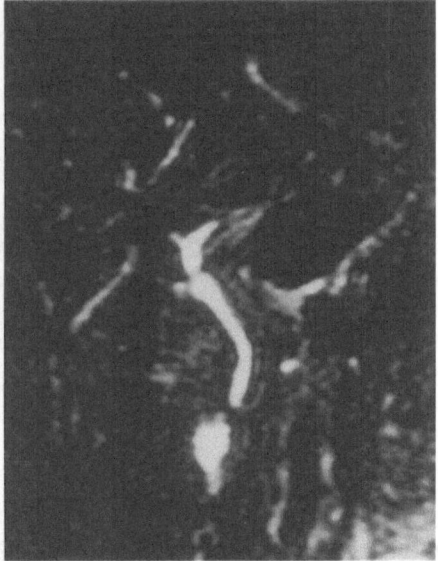

a                                                                                                   b

**Fig. 4. a** Smooth narrowing of the distal tract of the CBD, clear on MIP-reconstructed image. **b** At the confluence of the cystic duct an area of relative stenosis is evident on the
source image

formed by this approach. In four cases sphincterotomy had to be performed
after endoscopic.

In 12 cases dilatation of the bile ducts was present, with size ranging from
12 to 15 mm. No stones was evident in this group of patients and the dilatation was considered caused by papillary inflamation. In 2 cases axial slices
showed a thickening of the papilla, suggestive for this diagnosis. Due to the
presence of recurrent symptoms, sphyncterotomy through ERCP was performed in 4 this patients, while 5 patients with mild symptoms were fol-

**Fig. 5.** A significant stenosis at the level of the cystic duct confluence is evident on MRCP MIP-reconstructed (**a**) and source image (**b**)

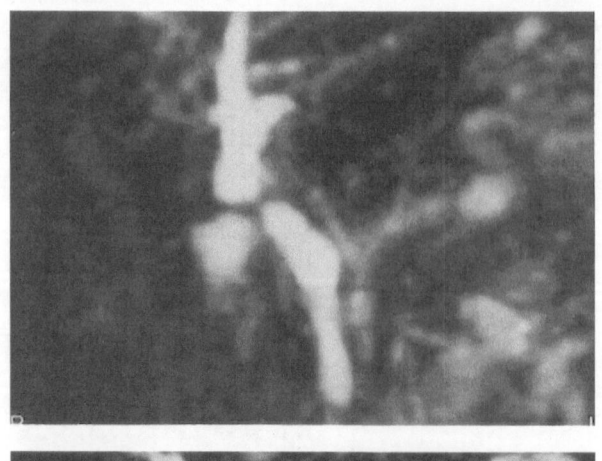

a

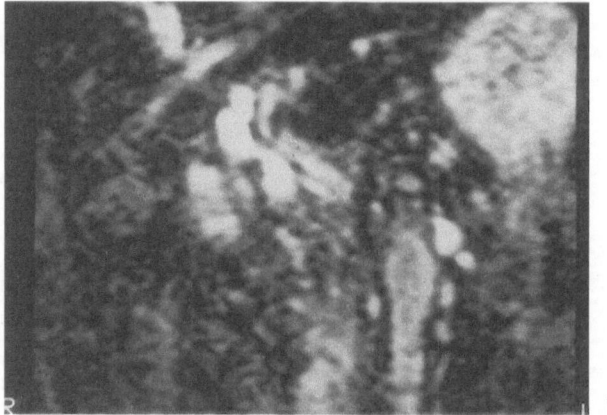

b

lowed up clinically. In three cases a peculiar finding was discovered. At the confluence of the cystic duct an area of relative stenosis was evident, better evaluated on the single slices of the acquisition. A clinical follow-up was undertaken in these three patients, due to the mildness of the symptoms.

Twelve patients had significant stenosis at the level of the cystic duct confluence. In seven there was residual lumen at the level of the stenosis in the analysis of single slices, and this finding was confirmed at subsequent ERCP (*n*=4) or percutaneous transhepatic biliary drainage (PTBD) (*n*=3). In five cases there was a complete absence of signal in the area of the lesion, without bile signal. In three of these cases PTBD performed afterwards showed the presence of residual lumen, with overstimation by MRCP. In two cases PTBD confirmed the diagnosis of complete obstruction.

In one case the fibrosis had extended to completely separate the right, and left duct system and percutaneous treatment with double approach was performed.

## Discussion

Laparoscopic cholecystectomy is currently the accepted procedure for treatment of gallbladder stones. Despite being a minimally invasive surgical procedure, complications may occur. These are generally related to the development of fibrosis at the level of the confluence of the cystic duct. Dilatation of the stenosis and placement of temporary stents by an endoscopic or percutaneous approach is the indicated treatment for these benign iatrogenic stenosis. Imaging of the bile ducts and evaluation of the stenosis is currently performed as the initial part of the therapeutic procedure.

Complications following surgery are not the only cause of symptoms in patients undergoing laparoscopic cholecystectomy. Symptoms may be due to the presence of recurrent stones or to inflammatory changes at the level of the papilla or may have no morphological background and result only from functional alteration in bile flow. Therefore a valid noninvasive imaging procedure is needed for screening patients to undergo invasive procedures and for determining the appropriate approach, whether percutaneous or endoscopic. Our experience shows that MRCP can be considered a valid procedure for the noninvasive evaluation of this group of patients.

In our experience ten patients presented with normal findings. Mild symptoms following removal of the gallbladder were well known even before the application of the new surgical procedures [9]. These symptoms often have no morphological cause. The bile ducts present normal size, there is no evidence of morphological alteration at the level of the papilla, and no residual stones are found. In this group of patients only follow-up must be performed. The value of MRCP is particularly evident in these patients since only a relatively invasive procedure could provide clues for diagnosis, considering the poor performance of intravenous cholangiography and also the fact that manufacturers have removed cholagiographic contrast medium from the market in many European countries due to the high cost of production and restricted indications for the procedure. Among the causes of the symptoms are functional disturbances to bile flow. If symptoms persist in these patients, a functional study must be perfomed. Manometric evaluation of the bile ducts has been proposed and is currently performed in selected instances [10]. Depending on the results of the manometric studies, sphyncterotomy may be indicated. Although in our series sphyncterotomy was never performed among such patients, we believe that MRCP allows restriction of the indications to sphyncterotomy only to patients really in need for this procedure.

CBD stones are present in 5%–10% of patients with gallbladder stones [11]. Preoperative identification of main bile duts stones can be achieved in 50%–70% of patients by using ultrasound [12]). Intravenous cholangiography is no longer perfomed, and therefore many patients undergo gallbladder removal without a correct preoperative diagnosis of CBD stones. Opinions in the literature differ as to the best procedure for treating these patients. Some surgeons routinely perform intraoperative cholangiography followed by removal of the CBD stones by a transcystic or transcholedochal approach [13].

Other surgeons prefer not to perform intraoperative cholangiography and perform endoscopic removal of CBD stones following surgery in cases with positive symptoms. In our series we evaluated various groups of patients undergoing gallbladder surgery. No CBD stones were found in those in whom intraoperative cholangiography had been performed.

The stones were evident on MIP images in only four cases, while in the remaining cases the stones could be shown in the single slices. A careful evaluation of each slice acquired on MRCP must be performed in identifying CBD stones, as shown in previous series. MRCP in these patients allowed a noninvasive evaluation to screen for patients to undergo endoscopic removal of stones. It is relevant that the symptoms of patients with stones did not differ from those of patients without significant morphological findings and mild symptoms (nausea, vomiting, residual colic, and general discomfort) or from those with bile duct stenosis and severe symptoms (jaundice and colics). MRCP is therefore a valid screening procedure also in this group of patients.

Dilatation of the bile ducts is a common finding following cholecystectomy. Without the presence of significant symptoms, dilatation of the bile ducts is considered part of the postoperative findings. In 12 of our patients there was dilatation of bile ducts of 12–15 mm. A morphological cause of the dilatation may exist, related to papillary phlogosis, or a functional cause, related to bile duct flow alteration. In either case MRCP is able to define the anatomy of the bile ducts and to exclude other causes of symptoms, such as stones and iatrogenic stenosis. In two cases of our series we also detected a thickening of the papilla due to inflammatory changes. The decision to perform therapeutic sphyncterotomy is made upon the importance of the symptoms. In our cases with bile duct dilatation sphyncterotomy was performed following MRCP in only four of nine patients. Again, the advantage of MRCP in screening for these patients and the importance of the symptoms in defining the cases to undergo ERCP and sphyncterotomy is evident in our series.

There was a very peculiar finding in three patients of our series, each of whom had mild symptoms following surgery. On MRCP no evidence of morphological alteration was evident in the MIP-reconstructed images, and there was only minimal dilatation of the bile ducts. However, the evaluation of single slices showed an area of relative reduction in size on the marginal slices (anterior in two cases and posterior in one case). These stenosis were considered clinically insignificant due to the minimal symptoms present in these patients. To our knowledge, this is the first time that minimal stenosis following cholecystectomy has been shown morphologically. In our cases, due to mild symptoms, ERCP could not be performed for lack of consent by the patients. We presume that these patients, since they reported symptoms related to heavy meals, suffer symptoms only in cases of stress for the bile system, with increase in relative flow. It will be interesting to follow-up these patients over the years to determine whether they develop significant symptoms.

Stenosis of the bile ducts following cholecystectomy is one of the most feared complications of biliary surgery. Its incidence has increased due to the use of laparoscopy, and the role of surgeon experience is evident [13, 14]. In the presence of iatrogenic stenosis symptoms may vary from increasing jaundice, to cholestasis without jaundice (increased phosphatases alkaline), to mild symptoms or recurrent colics. A noninvasive procedure to evaluate the biliary tree has the goal of screening for patients with stenosis to undergo interventional procedure and to provide an anatomic evaluation of the biliary tree and of the extension of the stenosis to define the most correct approach for treatment, by either transhepatic or endoscopic approach.

In 12 cases we correctly demostrated iatrogenic stenosis following laparoscopic cholecystectomy. The stenosis was present at the level of the confluence of the cystic duct in 11 patients, while in one there was a large fibrotic reaction, with complete extension to the confluence of the hepatic ducts and complete separation of the right and left bile duct systems.

In conclusion, MRCP has been shown to provide valid results in evaluating patients presenting symptoms following laparoscoic cholecystectomy. The various symptoms presented by these patients are not correlated with morphological findings. It is well known that dyspeptic symptoms are more often related to nonbiliary digestive pathology (e.g., gastritis, colitis). Therefore MRCP is the ideal noninvasive procedure for differentiating the cases not to undergo any intervention from those requiring intervention either for endoscopic removal of stones or sphyncterotomy or for dilatation of iatrogenic stenosis. Mapping the anatomy of the biliary tree is also helpful for defining the best approach in treating iatrogenic stenosis, either by transhepatic or endoscopic approach. The noninvasiveness of MRCP is important both to patients and to surgeons, considering the medicolegal implication that complications following this type of surgery may have.

## References

1. National Center for Health Statistic (1987) Summary: national hospital discharge survey. In: Advance data from vital and health statistics, no 159. National Center for Statistics, Hyattsville (DHHS publication no 88–1250)
2. NHI Consensus Conference (1993) Gallstones and laparoscopic cholecystectomy. JAMA 269(8):1018
3. Cuschieri A, Dubois F, Mouiel J, Mouret P, Becker H, Buess G, Trede M, Troidl H (1991) The European experience with laparoscopic cholecystectomy. Am J Surg 161:385
4. Gedacz TR (1993) US experience with laparoscopic cholecystectomy. Am J Surg 165:450
5. Ponsky JL (1991) Complications of laparoscopic cholecystectomy. Am J Surg 161:393
6. Harvey RB Hartman W (1993) Complications after laparoscopic cholecystectomy. Am J Surg 165:533
7. Wright TB, Bertino RB, Bishop AF et al (1993) Complications of laparoscopic cholecystectomy and their interventional radiologic management. Radiographics 13:119–128
8. Hunter J (1991) Avoidance of bile duct injury during laparoscopic cholecistectomy. Am J Surg 162:71
9. Speranza V (1991) Surgical treatment of extrahepatic stones. Changing concepts in biliary stones. Management Problems Gen Surg 8:283
10. De Masi E, Corazziari E, Mobih et al (1984) Manometric study of the sphinter of Oddi in patients with and without common bile duct stones. Gut 25:275
11. Hermann R (1991) The spectrum of biliary stone disease. Am J Surg 161:171–173
12. Pasanen P, Partanen K, Pikkarainen P, Alhava E, Pirinen A, Janatuinen E (1992) Ultrasonography, CT and ERCP in the diagnosis of choledochal stones. Acta Radiologica 33:53–56

12. Leroche E, Paganini A, Lomanto A et al (1996) Laparoscopic treatment of galldbladder and common bile duct stones: World J Surg (in press)
13. Hunter JG (1991) Avoidance of bile duct injury during laparoscopic cholecystectomy. Am J Surg 162:71–76
14. Ress AM, Sarr MG, Nagormy DM et al (1993) Spectrum and managment of mayor complications of laparoscopic cholecystectomy. Am J Surg 165:655–669

# Does MRCP Improve the Diagnosis of Pancreatic Pathologies?

## Introduction

Diagnostic evaluation of pancreatic diseases is based primarily on ultrasound and CT morphological findings. Such diseases as chronic pancreatitis, stones, pseudocysts, and in some cases pancreatic neoplsms can be characterized only in association with study of the pancreatic parenchyma and evaluation of the pancreatic duct. No contrast agent is excreted by the pancreas; therefore opacification of the pancreatic duct was achieved until recently only by direct contrast agent injection with ERCP. However, cannulation of the pancreatic duct is not possible in all cases, and some risks are related to this invasive procedure.

MRI provides morphological images of the pancreas by means of T1- and T2-weighted images. Its accuracy in staging pancreatic neoplasms is reported to be similar to that of CT [1]. Scattered reports have appeared on the use of MRI in the evaluation of chronic pancreatitis. However, reduced spatial resolution and the lack of evidence of calcifications has until now limited the potential diagnostic role of MRI in this field.

MRCP has recently been proposed for imaging both biliary and pancreatic ducts. Various pulse sequences can be employed with the same aim: to obtain a very high signal of the stationary fluids, canceling at the same time the signal of surrounding solid tissues. Both heavily T2-weighted turbo spin echo sequences and steady-state free precession sequences can be employed. Depending on the technique employed, breath-hold or non-breath-hold examinations can be carried out. The latter must be associated with respiratory compensation techniques.

Soto [2] and Takehara [3] have confirmed the value of MRCP in visualizing pancreatic duct abnormalities. Each of these series used high-field systems. Most equipment in Europe is currently of medium-field systems. Newer systems with high gradient strength (over 15 mT/m) provide the possibility of acquiring images with turbo spin echo techniques, using long echo times and long echo train length.

We optimized a non-breath hold 3D turbo spin echo MRCP sequence for visualizating the pancreatic duct. The sequence was used as a first diagnostic procedure in association with morphological T1- and T2-weighted spin echo sequences in patients with pancreatic pathology. The aim of the study was to compare the diagnostic value of MRCP to that of MRI in pancreatic pathology to determine the types of cases in which this technique could replace CT and ERCP.

## Personal Series

In the period from January 1995 to January 1996 a total of 63 consecutive patients (41 male, 22 female; ranging in age from 20 to 82 years; mean age 57.4 years) underwent MRI for evaluation of pancreatic pathology. All had been referred by the gastroenterological or surgical department to the radiological department for evaluation of suspected pancreatic pathology, based on clinical and ultrasound findings. The ultrasound data were not known when MRI was performed. The final diagnoses, obtained at surgery in 21 cases, at ERCP/PTC in 15 cases, at CT in 11 cases, and at follow-up in 16 cases, were: pancreatic carcinoma, 39; pancreatitis, 19; duodenal carcinoma, 2; and ampullary tumor, 3.

In this work only flogistic and neoplastic pancreatic diseases have been considered, thus excluding the three cases of ampullary tumors and the two cases of duodenal carcinoma.

ERCP and PTC procedures were performed in 15 of 58 patients (13 ERCP and 2 PTC), with interventional indication in nine and for further diagnostic evaluation in six. In three the pancreatic duct could not be filled by ERCP because of anatomic or techincal difficulties. CT was perfomed in 11 cases following MRI (third-generation equipment, CT Pace, GE Medical, Milwaukee, WI, USA). Contiguous 8-mm- thick slices were acquired before and after contrast agent injection. An automatic injector was employed (Medrad, etc.) to perform a biphasic injection: a bolus of 50 ml at 3 ml/s, followed by an infusion of 100 ml at 1 ml/s. Nonionic contrast agent was employed in every case at 300 mgI/ml concentration (Iomeprol, Bracco, Milan, Italy).

### Image Analysis

MR images were analyzed prospectively by two of the authors (P.P., A.L.). The cases were evaluated immediately after performing MRI. Both MIP reconstruction and source images of the MRCP sequence were available. In addition to defining the morphological findings, they were asked also to consult with the enoscopist, and together they decided whether to perform ERCP following MRCP. Image quality, parenchymal alteration (masses, atrophy, gross calcification), visualization of the pancreatic duct, size of the duct, presence of stenosis, and intraluminal defects were evaluated.

### Results

#### Image Quality

MRI images were of optimal quality in all of the cases. MRCP provided images of optimal quality in 43 (68%) and good in 20 (32%). Poor quality of the images was not related to significant motion artifacts in any patients, even uncooperative ones. Similarly, poor quality of the images did not impair the diagnostic value of the procedure in any patients.

### Parenchymal Alterations

*Focal Pancreatic Masses.* Focal pancreatic masses were present in 52 patients (82.5): 39 cases of adenocarcinomas, eight of focal chronic pancreatitis, three ampullary tumors, and two duodenal carcinomas. The lesions were in all cases clearer in T1-weighted images, while intrinsic contrast was limited in T2-weighted images. Lesion size averaged 3.7 cm (range 1.5–6 cm).

In 43 cases the MRI diagnosis was pancreatic cancer, and in four focal chronic pancreatitis, based on the presence of gross calcifications, detected as very low signal intensity lesions on T1- and T2-weighted images. No cases of focal chronic pancreatitis (15) were misdiagnosed as cancer. However, three cases at surgery and one at clinical follow-up (patient refused surgery) proved to be areas of focal chronic pancreatitis. In all these cases, there was a small hypointense lesion in the head of the pancreas, without infiltration of the peripancreatic fat, with morphological features similar to those of pancreatic cancer. The resulting sensitivity was 100%, specificity 78.9%, positive predictive value 90.6, negative predictive value 100%, and diagnostic accuray 93.1%.

*Diffuse Areas of Signal Intensity Changes.* Diffuse parenchymal alterations were evident in 12/19 cases (63.1%). There were diffuse patchy areas of hypointensity, evident on T1-weighted images. In T2-weighted images the signal intensity was generally inhomogeneus, but the definition of areas of parenchymal alteration was not as evident as in T1-weighted images. The finding was considered compatible with chronic pancreatitis, and depending on the clinical findings no further diagnostic modalities were performed. In two cases ERCP was performed to further define the pathology, with the aim of performing interventional procedures.

*Parenchymal Atrophy.* A total of 16/19 patients presented a marked reduction in pancreatic parenchyma. The atrophy was diffuse to all the body in twelve cases and was related to diffuse chronic pancreatitis. In these cases the reduction in parenchyma corresponded to low signal intensity of the residual parenchyma, a finding consistent with chronic pancreatitis. In four cases the atrophy was limited to the tail region due to occlusion of the pancreatic duct related to tumor in one case, focal chronic pain in one, and pseudocysts in two. No further diagnostic procedure was performed in this group of patients.

*Pseudocysts.* Pseudocysts were present in weven patients (11%). In five there were multiple cysts. The diameter ranged between 0.8 cm and 12 cm (mean 5.3 cm)

In four cases there was clear contact with the pancreatic duct, also evident in the source images. This finding was considered suggestive for communication with the duct. In five patients ERCP was performed that discovered communication with the duct, not evident in MRCP in two other patients.

### Bile Duct Involvement

*Visualization of the Common Bile Duct.* The bile ducts were normal in 26 patients. Bile ducts were dilated in 32 cases, with marked dilatation in 14 (duct size over 15 mm). In normally sized bile ducts, full evidence of the CBD was obtained in 10 cases, with only partial visualization in six.

### Pancreatic Duct Involvement

*Visualization of the Pancreatic Duct.* The pancreatic duct was fully visualized in 51 patients (81%) with concomitant visualization of the accessory duct in four cases (6.3%). In seven of the patients (14%), the Wirsung duct was normal. In the remaining 44 cases, the Wirsung duct was dilated: 2–4 mm in 21 cases (33%) and more than 4 mm in 23 (36.5%). In 13 cases (21%), secondary ducts were visualized. A beaded appearance was present in six cases (36%) of chronic pancreatitis, while a homogeneous dilation was evident in 24 cases (41.4%).

*Stenosis.* Duct strictures were present in 23 cases. In 16 cases the stricture was single and located in the head of the pancreas, due to a focal mass in the head of the pancreas. In two cases there was a stricture in the body-tail of the pancreas, and in five there were multiple strictures, alternating with dilatation of the duct, with a beaded appearance. ERCP confirmed the stenotic involvement of the duct in the cases in which it was performed. MRCP slightly overestimated the stenosis in two of five cases of chronic pancreatitis with single or multiple stenosis.

*Filling Defects.* In six cases there were filling defects due to stones, single in two and multiple in four. The stones were evident in the MIP images in one of six patients, while the source images the stones could be determined in the remaining patients only after careful evaluation of. ERCP was performed in all cases for interventional purpose to confirm the diagnosis. A further case with panceatic pseuodcyst showed the presence of a impacted stone in the distal part of the stone, which as evident on MRCP source images only after careful retrospective evalution.

### MRCP Improvement

In eight cases (20.5%) with pancreatic carcinoma and in 12 cases (63%) with chronic pancreatitis, MRCP findings improved the diagnostic value of conventional MRI.

## Pseudocysts

In ten patients MRCP showed saccular dilatation adjacent to the pancreatic duct, due to pseudocysts; these were 0.5–10 cm in size. In two there was clear contact with the pancreatic duct, also evident in the source images. This finding was suggested communication with the duct. In six patients ERCP was performed, and in two it revealed discovered communication with the duct not evident in MRCP. In four cases no ERCP was performed, and the patients underwent immediate surgical drainage of the pseudocyst.

## Discussion

Our series shows that MRI supported by MRCP sequences is highly accurate in determining pancreatic pathology. MRCP improved the diagnostic yield of MRI in all cases with biliary or pancreatic ducts involvement. This was important in neoplastic cases, but the improvement was evident particularly in patients with chronic pancreatitis. In this group of patients MRCP allowed complete and detailed anatomic evaluation of the pancreatic duct involvement, showing patterns similar to those on ERCP. The overlap of findings obtained with the two procedures was such that ERCP was considered to provide no further diagnostic information, and its use was limited mostly to interventional procedures. The only advantage of ERCP was in determining the communication of pseudocysts with the pancreatic duct, a finding not provided by MRCP.

At our insititution we began using MRCP over 1 year ago. In this period the confidence of the referring physicians and of the radiologists has grown to such an extent that MRCP is now the first diagnostic procedure to be performed in evaluating patients with suspected pancreatic pathology (with the exception of acute pancreatitis). The results obtained are positive, and the use of other diagnostic procedures following MRI is limited.

From a cost-effective point of view, this saves in expenditure. We replace two procedures commonly usually performed in this field (CT and ERCP) by single procedure (MRI with MRCP). CT should be used only in rare cases, principally when calcifications are suspected on MRI and need to be verified by CT. ERCP will retain an important role only for interventional procedures. However, many patients undergo immediate surgical intervention without the need for preoperative endoscopic intervention. It is our feeling that in many cases endoscopists place biliary stents even in patients who are potential surgical candidates. The use of MRI to determine the indications for treatment (surgical or endoscopic) will limit the number of stents to be placed.

## References

1. Megibow AJ, Zhou XH, Rotterdam H, Francis IR, Zerhouni EA, Balfe DM, Weinreb JC, Aisen A, Kuhlman J, Heiken JP et al (1995) Pancreatic adenocarcinoma: CT versus MR imaging in the evaluation of resectability–report of the Radiology Diagnostic Oncology Group. Radiology 195:327–332

2. Soto JA, Barish MA, Yucel EK, Clarke P, Siegenberg D, Chuttani R, Ferrucci JT (1995) Pancreatic duct: MR cholangiopancreatography with a three dimensional fast spin echo technique. Radiology 196: 459–464
3. Takehara Y, Ichijo K, Tooyama N, Kodaira N et al (1994) Breath-hold MR cholangio-pancreatography with a long echo train fast spin echo sequence and a surface coil in chronic pancreatitis. Radiology 192:73–78

# Subject Index